Blue Cross
Since 1929:
Accountability
and the Public Trust

Blue Cross Since 1929: Accountability and the Public Trust

Odin W. Anderson

Ballinger Publishing Company ● **Cambridge, Mass.** *1975*
A Subsidiary of J.B. Lippincott Company

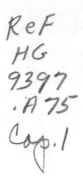

International Standard Book Number: 0–88410–122–3

Library of Congress Catalog Card Number: 74–32003

Printed in the United States of America

Library of Congress Cataloging in Publication Data

Anderson, Odin Waldemar, 1914–
   Blue Cross since 1929: a study in public accountability.

   Bibliography: p.
   1. Blue Cross Association—History. I. Title. [DNLM: 1. Insurance, Health—History—United States. 2. Insurance, Hospitalization—History—United States. W275 AA1 A57b]
HG9397.A75   368.3'8'00973   74–32003
ISBN 0–88410–122–3

Contents

Preface and Acknowledgements

The opportunity to shape a general line of investigation is a privilege. In this book on the Blue Cross idea, I attempt to deepen my long-standing interest in the development of health services delivery and financial systems in the United States and abroad by dealing largely with one financing agency for hospital care and its interrelationships with the private and public sectors. The Blue Cross system is an interesting and significant example of the role of the private sector in health services and its relationship to government funding.

I was approached by Walter J. McNerney, President, Blue Cross Association, in 1970, to undertake a history of the Blue Cross development. His conditions were in the best academic tradition, that this would be my project and my book. It was not to be an official history of the Blue Cross idea. One specific condition, however, was most welcome, because I might not have thought it feasible. This was that I should interview the pioneers of the movement, who are scattered all over the country, almost all in retirement. It was suggested that I should compile a set of tapes or oral histories for the record. This has been a most gratifying task. I have interviewed all starters of Blue Cross plans who were alive during my fieldwork and taped their recollections and remarks for a couple of hours each. They were informative, cooperative, and congenial. It was reassuring to learn first hand that Blue Cross plans were started by essentially public spirited and decent people. They were a surprisingly happy lot in that they would "do it all over again," and they felt that they had made contributions to their communities.

The Blue Cross Association provided an ample budget for this project and gave me unconditional access to association records and meetings, including executive sessions. The travel entailed was extensive, as can be seen by my notes of the places all over the country where I interviewed the pioneers.

Specific acknowledgements go to Frank Morn, a graduate student in American history at the University of Chicago, and to Robin Boger, a graduate student in business, economics, and education, also at the University of Chicago, for helping me gather data. Elaine Scheye at the Center for Health Administration Studies was helpful in editing the first draft. Robert M. Cunningham, recently retired as editor of *Modern Hospital*, improved the final draft of the manuscript considerably. I wish to thank Antone Singsen at the Blue Cross Association for being my helpful coordinator in that agency, and his secretary, Eunice Foskett. Finally, I wish to thank Evelyn Friedman, my secretary, for the endless clerical assistance a book entails.

Odin W. Anderson, Ph.D.
Chicago
November 4, 1974

Chapter One

Introduction

The development of Blue Cross hospital plans was clearly a social movement, because there was a perceived problem: the high cost episodes of hospital care for families over a given period, and depleted hospital financing. Also there was a latent division of labor, which a social movement needs—a theoretician, or idea man, a promoter, an organizer, and a potential corps of action-oriented people who catch fire when they encounter the idea man, the promoter, and the organizer. In due course, a self-determined group is formed, linking up with other groups and interests, a prime characteristic of American society. Some start-up capital is found, and official sanction is sought.

If the concept is sound and the leadership adequate, the movement is on its way. If the concept is unsound, behind the times, or ahead of its time, any leadership will fail. If the concept is an expression of an idea "whose time has come," it will succeed even under barely adequate leadership, and it will succeed brilliantly under brilliant leadership. By all standards, the Blue Cross movement has been a success, whether brilliant or not is left to the judgment of others, but success is undeniable. Whether or not it could or should have been more successful, according to its own objectives, is still another question, since all social enterprises are assumed to be able to accomplish more than they do.

The continuing success of the Blue Cross system will be tested in terms of circumstances, objectives and countervailing forces in which it is now heavily engaged. Its leadership will have to feel congenial with social, economic, and political complexities of the age we live in. Such leadership will need a variety of talents, as was true of the early leaders—theoreticians, promoters, organizers, and technicians who know how to roll with the punches. The Blue

Cross idea has emerged as the most influential latent force in the private sector of the health field to counterbalance other single, powerful forces among the providers of service—hospitals and physicians—and their respective organizations, private insurance companies, and the federal government. Thus, Blue Cross development may serve as a case study of private and public interrelationships, a problem very much under discussion these days in all sectors of the economy. Blue Cross plans became the first large-scale financing mechanism for hospital care, particularly in voluntary hospitals, for middle and lower middle income groups. Blue Cross plans became a reference point for later developments in health care financing—medical society-sponsored physician prepayment plans, soon to be called Blue Shield (the same color symbolizing the linkage but appropriately with different insignia), and the private insurance companies. The early success of Blue Cross plans created emulators and competitors.

In a substantial sense this case study is a history of the Blue Cross movement; but it is not a history in the traditional sense of meticulous attention to a chronology of events, dates, specific persons, and Blue Cross plans. What is intended instead is a description of the effort to coordinate Blue Cross plans into both local and national entities in order to cope with local differences and needs and national uniformities simultaneously. Accordingly, judgments will have to be made constantly as to emphasis, attributions of influence, and origins.

One of the risks of writing recent history is that almost all the people who feel closely identified with the origins and development of a movement may still be alive, informed within their own spheres, and understandably sensitive. Indeed, a novel attribute of this study is that the histories were obtained largely from personal interviews with many of the early leaders in Blue Cross (see Appendix A). They were asked to recall the circumstances that opened the way to Blue Cross development, early problems, major issues they faced in the 25 years or more they were associated with the movement, and personal anecdotes. The content of these interviews provides an invaluable store of information, insights, and atmosphere which are not usually found in minutes of meetings, official documents, and annual reports, or in local Blue Cross histories, of which there are a few (see Appendix C).

In addition to the personal interviews, the factual history of Blue Cross plans and related prepayment and insurance agencies is presented in brief to show the pace of growth, enrollment and financial, and the major events shaping the whole health care and health insurance enterprise. These facts and events are a matter of record, and they have been consulted exhaustively, but are presented selectively.

I have been observing the health care field in general, and voluntary health insurance in particular, for 30 years. I know personally the leaders in all sectors of the health care enterprise and have followed the events that will be described; in some instances I have observed them at first hand. My primary and constant interest has been the relationship of health care delivery systems and financing methods to the environing social, economic, and political context.

In view of the fact that this study will be highly interpretive, although based on facts wherever possible, and on careful inferences, it will necessarily reflect my own personal predilections and analytical style. It will present a point of view as to the nature of American society, the nature of the health services enterprise, the possibilities for equitable access to health care on the part of the public, and the context in which health care delivery systems and their funding can remain dynamic—all this with reference to the public interest and public accountability.

Chapter Two

Pluralism: Safety in Numbers

The Blue Cross system is a distinctly American institution which grew out of the nonprofit fraction of the private sector, stemming from the nonprofit character of the voluntary hospitals. Whatever function the nonprofit sector may have in the health field, as well as in other endeavors, the persistence of the nonprofit concept is impressive. In the health field, the nonprofit sector may well be a bridge between the private, for-profit sector and the government.

Some evidence that this is the case may be found in a statement on national policy by the Committee for Economic Development, the prestigious organization financed by many American businesses to sponsor research in economic policy

> The great growth of corporations in size, market power, and impact on society has naturally brought with it a commensurate growth in responsibilities; in a democratic society, power sooner or later begets equivalent accountability.
>
> Current profitability, once regarded as the dominant if not exclusive objective, is now often seen more as a vital means and powerful motivating force for achieving broader ends, rather than as an end in itself.
>
> The modern professional manager . . . regards himself, not as an owner disposing of personal property as he sees fit, but as a trustee balancing the interests of many diverse participants and constituents in the enterprise, whose interests sometimes conflict with others.[1]

[1]Committee for Economic Development, Research and Policy Committee, *Social Responsibilities of Business Corporations; A Statement on National Policy* (New York: 1971), pp. 12, 22. In the same vein and revealing growing concern with the social responsibility of corporations: Paul T. Heyne, *Private Keepers of the Public Interest* (New York: McGraw-Hill, 1968); Neil H. Jacoby, *Corporate Power and Social Responsibility; A Blueprint for the Future* (New York: MacMillian, 1973); Phillip I. Blumberg, "The Politicization of the Corporation," *The Business Lawyer* July, 1971, pp. 1551–1587.

This would seem to be an idealized version of the modern manager and a model for Blue Cross directors.

As a reaction to disenchantment with reliance on government for solutions, since 1966 Harris polls have revealed that the American public has escalated its expectations of business leadership. The reason for this expectation has been that bankers and businessmen are seen as "having the money and the clout to get things done." Harris is of the opinion that for the business community, this change in attitude "could be an opportunity to reassert its role of leadership in a new and different way from the past. Instead of being an adjunct of a GOP regime, business leaders could now be an independent force, pressing for positive change in society, setting a new kind of example. The public mandate was there."[2]

Although government is the ultimate repository of the public interest, it also needs to be watched and held accountable as severely as any other sector. No sector has a monopoly on virtue or competence. If there is in the body politic enough political sophistication to appreciate the value of tension between the private and public sectors in the financing and provision of health services, this country will be able to develop a variety of health delivery systems in relation to its geographic, economic, and population diversities. If there is not enough political sophistication to encourage and tolerate such diversities, we shall then settle for the lowest common denominator commensurate with that level of political timidity.

In this country the government does not own the mainstream of health service facilities, nor are the health professionals public functionaries on salaries. The backbone of the hospital system is the voluntary hospital; the backbone of the health professions is private practice. There is no likelihood in the foreseeable future that the hospitals will be expropriated or that health professionals will be made public functionaries. This is so because Congress is chary of having the government own anything if the public can be served some other way, such as by contract, or by applying regulation, financial incentives, and various kinds of leverages. What then follows is that in the event of universal health insurance the government will probably contract in some way with providers or their representatives in order to carry out the mandate of the insurance legislation. There are many precedents for this, since modern governments of the liberal-democratic model are mandated to assure an increasing flow of goods and services. There are various ways governments can do this. In all liberal-democratic countries, a common method has been contracting out rather than setting up government-owned industries. In fact, so

---

[2] Louis Harris, *The Anguish of Change* (New York: Norton, 1973). pp. 161–162, 164–165.

extensive is the use of the administrative contract in this country, and to a lesser extent in Great Britain, that one political scientist coined the term "the contract state" to characterize modern governments.[3]

In the health services the contract relationship is a particularly difficult one, because there is a paucity of performance indicators which can be specified in the contract so that the contracting parties know what they are selling and buying. In some other areas for contracting out, specifications can be worked out, as with contractors who build highways and must meet standards of cement mix, width, thickness, and length, or in the more highly technical products of a moonshot.

An underlying assumption behind contracting out is that government does not have the organization and the appropriate personnel to undertake large enterprises under its own ownership and control, or that it would be a wasteful duplication for government to set up the organization and personnel if these already exist and government can contract with them, or that possibly the private sector can operate with more flexibility and perhaps more efficiency than government. A final assumption, which may be the most important (and least discussed), is that contracting out diffuses power in the body politic, avoiding extreme centralization of authority and funding.

The presumption underlying the contracting out concept is that government is given access to a vast organizational and technical resource in which the contractor and government can work as honest adversaries. The contractors are at risk. The entire health economy is thereby invigorated. If government controls all mandated services, the presumption is that there will be relative inflexibility and rigidity. As Rufus Rorem, an early Blue Cross leader who had a prominent part in this history, said some years ago: "The essence of government is not quality but equity; certainty, right down the line. That is a very important distinction. It isn't originality, but certainty."[4] The mandated services can be contracted out, but there can also be services which are not mandated and are covered by private agencies. Very seldom have governments been willing or able to offer a complete health service virtually free of charge at time of service, on the National Health Service model of Great Britain. There is always room for supplemental benefits, exploration of new services, and experiments with innovations in delivery methods. A judicious combination of the public and private sectors will assure a dynamism that is seemingly more difficult to achieve in a purely governmental operation.

[3]Bruce L. R. Smith, "Accountability and Independent in the Contract State," in *The Dilemma of Accountability in Modern Government; Independence Versus Contract*, Bruce L. R. Smith and D. C. Hague eds. (New York: St. Martin's Press, 1971), p. 3.
[4]Interview in New York, December 17, 1970.

The validity of the foregoing premises can be argued indefinitely.[5] Political philosophies are difficult to argue logically. Basically, one believes a given premise or one doesn't. The basic premise here is the fear of concentrated power. What is then desired is a structured adversary relationship between the parties at interest. A method of orderly and periodic confrontation must be evolved.

This concept is particularly appropriate to the health service delivery system. Although both the provision and financing of health services have become wholly a government responsibility in some western liberal-democratic countries, there would seem to be no inherent logic in government's being the primary providing or funding agency unless the overriding objective is an approximation of pure equity at the price of rigidity. An equally important objective, however, is a built-in mechanism to assure change. The structured adversary relationship will facilitate change. Given the great complexity of the health services, the difficulties of establishing specifications, and the personal nature of health care, no central body should be given the power to determine the shape of the health services delivery system and the general level of resources devoted to it.

This country is wise in the art of the possible, a concept that is frequently assumed to harbor cynicism. The height of cynicism, however, is to promise more than can be delivered or to deliver service in a form most of the people and providers of the service do not want. This is why a known range of options of delivery systems seems so desirable, with financing mandated by government by payroll deductions from employers and employees, and with generous subsidies for the low income population to buy into the mainstream of health services. Above a certain minimum income, the benefit package can be

---

[5] A recent publication which would take issue with these premises is Sylvia A. Law. *Blue Cross: What Went Wrong?* (New Haven: Yale University Press, 1974). The book clearly supports the prevailing view that health services and costs are in a "crisis" and that the self-evident solution is greater consumer control and participation in health services delivery. The chief scapegoat is the Blue Cross system because of its high visibility and its presumption, in the author's view, of carrying the mantle of the public interest. The book, however, is not a study of the Blue Cross system. It is equally a study of HEW and Medicare, the Civil Service Commission, the behavior of Congress, consumerism, and how to implement national health insurance. The entire health services delivery system is severly criticized and Blue Cross is a more convenient villan among other villains. The author boxes herself in completely. She distrusts Congress, HEW, Blue Cross, SSA, and even health maintenance organizations (the latter may have the incentive to cut costs at the expense of adequate service). She is then left with consumer control, which she also distrusts, and retreats by designating experts to be consumer advocates. She presents, therefore, no strategy, not even one of countervailing forces between the private and public sectors, as suggested here, because she believes the same interests control both. She then provides no practical guide to improve the system within the constraints of the society of which it is a part.

optional. The Federal Employees Health Benefits Program is an example of this range of options which has been in operation since 1960. The negotiating process that led up to this program was in the best American political tradition.[6] The operation of the program has been relatively smooth, considering rising costs.

Since no single method of delivery and paying for services so far devised has been sufficiently or uniformly acceptable to all groups at interest, the offering of a variety of options, and the opportunity to change from one option to another, will be a safety valve for dissatisfactions, which are inherently high in a service that touches both the pocketbooks and anxieties of all the people. Further, this approach embodies a concept of basic services to be paid for in part by the employer or by taxation; the citizen may then add what he wishes within the rather wide range of alternatives available—from first dollar coverage to high cost episodes only. The low income and poverty segment of the population subsidized by the government can be given choices too, a plausible way to avoid the institutionalization of a two class system of medical care.

The use of government financing power directly to influence the particular form a delivery method should assume is threatening, as is government exercise of direct financial controls on the methods of reimbursing providers of services, and on the volume of services. It seems preferable for the government to exercise cost controls through rate negotiations within which each of the various contractors can work out its benefit package and price, with benchmarks for cost comparisons over time. Benefit structures, accessibility, and use of services are related to one another. All three are related to rates, and simultaneously they influence enrollment and solvency of the health services delivery system. It would seem that this set of relationships constitutes a potentially workable control mechanism which is more sensitive to changes in the system and at the same time more acceptable to various concerned groups than a more direct and necessarily more arbitrary form of financial control. The government should facilitate competition among delivery methods by putting the purchasing power in the hands of the buyers.

The foregoing discussion, of course, has direct implications for the impending possibility of some form of universal health insurance and the relationship of the government to the private sector. There are many precedents. The relatively small-scale precedent is the Federal Employees Health Benefits Program. The large-scale precedent, amounting to a colossus, is Medicare and the

---

[6]Odin W. Anderson and J. Joel May, *The Federal Employees Health Benefits Program: 1961–1968; A Model for National Health Insurance?* Perspectives A9 (Chicago: Center for Health Administration Studies, University of Chicago, 1971).

use of the contract between the Social Security Administration and the Blue Cross Association as the prime contractor, with subcontracting Blue Cross plans making payment to hospitals, nursing homes, and physicians.

Curiously enough, there has been no thorough evaluation of the government-intermediary relationship. An attempt was made to do this by an agreement between the National Academy of Public Administration and the Social Security Administration.[7] The evaluation was at best a position paper. No intensive investigation was contemplated. The final report starts out with a strong admonition to the parties at interest but recommends that the contractual relationship between the contractors and the Social Security Administration should continue, providing some changes are made in that relationship. The admonition reads as follows:

> The use of the contractors to perform administrative functions in the Medicare program is a classic case of the continuation of a legislated public policy with inadequate public concern for its consequences (underscoring added). Medicare has been functioning for seven years, utilizing Blue Cross, Blue Shield, and commercial insurance companies, as intermediaries and carriers to pay for, and and to the extent provided for under the Act exercise, elements of control over the quality, cost, and frequency of services.[8]

Yet, from the inception of the program, according to the report, both the parties at interest and the public as a whole have not addressed the fundamental question of the appropriateness or effectiveness of the use of carriers and intermediaries: Can the private institutions be utilized effectively to provide public services in a program as complex and politically sensitive as the provision of health services to the aged? What are the administrative requirements which governmental agencies should establish to make such use appropriate and effective? These questions are important but difficult to answer definitively. The issue is mainly political and philosophical; hence it is an issue of the appropriateness of the use of intermediaries and virtually beyond statistical evaluation, given the absence of performance indicators for a health service program, no matter who administers it.

[7]The publications resulting from this contract are Bruce L. R. Smith and Neil Hollander, eds., *The Administration of Medicare: A Shared Responsibility* (Washington, D.C.: National Academy of Public Administration, 1973); National Academy of Public Administration, *Final Report of the Medicare Project Panel* (Washington, D.C.: June 30, 1973). Also, there was general examination of this problem at the 1973 National Health Forum sponsored by the National Health Council, *The Changing Role of the Public and Private Sectors in Health Care.* Report of the 1973 National Health Forum (New York: 1973). The writer had explored this problem in his seminars on Contemporary Problems and Issues in the Health Field at the University of Chicago.

[8]National Academy of Public Administration, *Final Report.*

The prevailing opinion, as stated by the National Academy report, is that "The first phase of the Medicare program was characterized by the 'magnificent' administrative job that was done by both S.S.A. and the contractors. The sheer magnitude of organizing so massive a national system in such a short time is a credit to both the public and private sectors. It reflected the consummate ability of S.S.A. to enroll beneficiaries, establish eligibility and implement legislation and of the contractors to administer a complex insurance system."[9] Given this generous compliment, what then are the current problems and issues in the contracting method?

The initial priority was to establish a system to pay bills, and this was done expeditiously. The preamble to the act read, for example, that there was to be no interference with the current operating and organizational arrangements of the prevailing health services delivery system. The primary control of use (and therefore cost stemming from use) and quality was through the cautionary mechanism of review of hospital admissions after a certain number of days to determine the appropriateness of continued hospitalization. It was essentially a device to persuade physicians to talk to each other and establish visible norms.

What remained untested, according to the National Academy, was the question of the long term viability of using private contractors to manage a health program. Naturally, the problem of management became apparent when the expeditious paying of bills was associated with rapidly rising costs. The contract mechanism was not really designed to manage the health services system. This question came up later, so the contract concept should not be blamed for not containing costs. The contractors so far have had only partial power to do so by themselves. The original intent of the Medicare Act was to pay for services on demand. The intent of Congress was fulfilled, but in due course there was a cost crisis.

In the face of rapidly rising costs there followed an "avalanche of controls designed to maintain the fiscal integrity of the system," according to the National Academy. The results were (1) an increase in the controls placed upon the contractors by SSA; (2) a general atmosphere wherein the contractors were willing, or forced by adverse cost publicity, to accept whatever level of control would enable them and the government to reduce costs; and (3) lack of time on the part of the contracting parties to attempt agreement on a long-term relationship. It appears to the National Academy that "in many respects the current Medicare administration is still operating on this basis," The increasing concern in the contractual relationship is the need to influence quality and cost, a cruel challenge to contractors, but unavoidable given the worry about rising costs.

[9] Ibid, p. 5.

The National Academy report makes the correct assumption that the relationships between the contractors and SSA cannot continue without SSA stiffening controls so that contractor organizations increasingly become an arm of government, with no more or less latitude than any such agency. Instead of a shared responsibility, there will be a dependency relationship, vitiating the creative purpose of the contract concept.

The recommendations of the National Academy seem reasonable enough, although the academy is fully cognizant of the fact that parties at interest need to work out their relationship so that a true partnership and honest adversary positions can evolve. The main ingredients, however, are mutual trust and the good faith of all parties. Without good faith, contracts are empty mechanisms where nervous adversaries argue over technicalities not central to the relationship.

According to the academy, some basic decisions will have to be made by SSA regarding (1) the establishment of standards of performance on the part of the contractors, emphasizing results rather than detailed regulations which interfere with the internal operations of the contractor; (2) the timing of the administrative policy process so that contractors can enter into discussions of process early in the formulation of administrative policy; (3) a sympathetic attitude toward the contract concept; and (4) an arrangement for the top managements to deal with each other personally. A final and exceedingly important recommendation was that SSA should coordinate its activities closely with other units of the executive branch which affect the contractual relationship. There have been instances when SSA was not aware of policy changes affecting the Medicare contract with the Blue Cross system.[10]

According to the academy, the contractors would also have to make some changes. They should (1) accept the idea of public accountability and disclosure necessitated by the expenditure of public funds; (2) regard themselves as agents of the public rather than the providers; (3) understand fully that SSA has overall and ultimate administrative responsibility for the program, including evaluation of contractor performance; and (4) appeal through the political system only in the most serious circumstances as they increase their role in policy determination at the administrative level of the government. Presumably, this final recommendation should also apply to SSA.

[10] Robert M. Ball, former commissioner of SSA, reported: "In the case of the dropping of the two percent (margin above negotiated costs for hospitals) a decision was made at the level of the secretary and the departmental budget office even prior to consultation with the Social Security Administration . . . and little if any account was taken of the possible damage that could be done to the long-range partnership between Medicare and the hospitals by such unilateral action by the government," "That Illusive Partnership" (Speech delivered before the Colorado Hospital Association, Aspen, Colorado, September 13, 1973).

The foregoing recommendations deal mainly with the political and administrative philosophies underpinning public accountability when the private and public sectors cooperate. Obviously, it will take some time for the parties to work out a relationship in which they will continue as equals in Medicare and possible future contractual relationships. In this connection, it may be useful to mention three kinds of accountability which need to be balanced, according to David Z. Robinson.[11] He distinguishes between fiscal program and process. *Fiscal accountability* is the easiest to monitor. In the auditor's sense, funds should be spent according to appropriate procedure, in the manner designated by law and the terms of the contract, and standard accounting procedures are observed. *Program accountability* involves the question of whether the government is actually getting the results it sought through the program. This presumes, of course, that the government knows what results it wants. In the case of Medicare, the first priority was that the aged should have easier access to health services by reducing the economic barrier. This Medicare did. Later, Congress sought cost containment. Finally, *process accountability* is concerned with the appropriateness of the procedures by which the enterprise is carried out, given the difficulties of measuring outcome by program accountability.

When government contracts for health services it is concerned with all three types of accountability. Given the nature of the product—i.e., difficulty in specifications—fiscal accountability is given priority because it is easy and obviously necessary; process accountability follows; and program accountability comes last. It is on program accountability that the main problem of cost control now rests. Whether program accountability can be resolved in a contract between the private and public sectors will continue to test both administrative and political sophistication.

There are so far no agreed on criteria of performance of contractors which can be guaranteed in advance to be politically acceptable. The performance indicators—speed of paying providers, the rapidity with which correspondence is answered, or even the percentage of the gross income that goes for administrative costs—are not the primary indicators. The primary problem is politically tolerable cost containment. There can probably be no future for the contracting principle unless there is more political and administrative sophistication about administering an essentially open-ended service. No method so far is in essence and by definition good enough. This is one reason voluntary health insurance has been found wanting everywhere it has existed—in Sweden, Great Britain, Canada, and other Commonwealth countries.

[11]David Z. Robinson, "Government Contracting for Academic Research: Accountability in the American Experience," in *The Dilemma of Public Accountability in Modern Government,* Bruce L. R. Smith and D. C. Hague eds. (New York: St. Martin's Press, 1971), p. 103-128.

Voluntary health insurance was declared inadequate even in Canada, where it was vigorous and flourishing. This is also why contracting out to intermediaries may not be politically feasible in the long run. Canada considered the possibility of using Blue Cross and Blue Shield contractors when it enacted its hospital service legislation in 1958 and its physicians' service legislation in 1969. The prevailing political opinion emerged that government, in order to be accountable, must administer the national health insurance program itself for the service mandated by legislation.[12] Costs rise, and benefits are considered inadequate, and the final repository of responsibility becomes government. After that there is no other place to go, and the health services settle down within that particular framework. Government does not necessarily do a better job—it might even do a worse one, but there is more assurance of equity, and the government can put an arbitrary lid on expenditures within politically tolerable limits of access and quality. These are what have been called "wicked" problems, as against what are seen as "benign" problems. Wicked problems are those for which there are no definitive solutions. Benign problems can be solved. Wicked problems are resolved, as it were, continually, but are lacking agreed on specifications as to what a solution is. There is a tendency to blame persons or parties at interest for failures rather than to recognize that wicked problems are continually being resolved and reopened in the tension of the political process.[13]

The height of sophistication would be for the private and public sectors to battle it out within the contracting principle and within a known choice of options, the Federal Employees Health Benefits Program being a model. But perhaps the contracting parties will get weary of constant renegotiations of the contract, year after year. Perhaps the government agencies do not really want an equal adversary who can stare them down on occasion, and legitimately. Perhaps the private sector is incapable of being an equal adversary.

Still, if creative working relationships between the private and public sectors can be evolved, a minimum of arbitrary control will be needed. It will mean that the political and economic model of American society set forth in Chapter 4, and the problem-solving styles inherent in that model, have validity. Certainly the American health services system will remain open and pluralistic enough for contractors and intermediaries to function for the foreseeable future. An alert private sector can be a salutary force in this context.

[12]Interviews with A. G. Blair, Edmonton, Alberta, March 19, 1972; Duncan Milbain, T. Ledwell Doyle, and Harold Brown, Montreal, Quebec, June 19, 1973; and Walter E. Cannon, Chicago, August 22, 1973.
[13]Horst W. J. Rittel and Melvin M. Webber, "Dilemmas in a General Theory of Planning," *Policy Sciences* 4 (1973): 155–169.

Chapter Three

The Seed Bed

The Blue Cross concept had many origins. In the early 1930s, its originators were aware that circumstances were appropriate to start some kind of hospital prepayment plan. If the American voluntary nonprofit community hospital had not been the backbone of the hospital delivery system—as it was then and has largely remained—the Blue Cross idea would not have been invented. If the private practice of medicine had not been the backbone of the medical delivery system, linked to the voluntary hospitals, Blue Shield plans would not have followed. No one was, or is, admitted to a hospital without the decision of a physician.

The basic characteristics of the prevailing health services delivery system emerged during the latter part of the nineteenth and early in the twentieth century, a period of tremendous economic and industrial development in a political environment of limited government and unlimited free enterprise spurred by the profit motive. The great economic expansion resulted in a relatively large middle income group able to sustain a range of goods and services in the private sector with minimal, and generally grudging, government intervention. The broad American middle class created by the expansion should not be regarded as a self-conscious class in the European sense. The American class system was much more open and fluid. In this connection the observations made by Wiebe seem reasonable:

> In part, the new middle class was a class only by courtesy of the historian's afterthought. Covering too wide a range to form a tightly knit group, it divided into two main categories. One included those with strong, professional aspirations in such fields as medicine, law, economics, administration, social work, and architecture. The

second comprised specialists in business, labor, and in agriculture awakening both to their distinctiveness and to their ties with similar people in the same occupation. In fact, consciousness of unique skills and functions, an awareness that came to mold much of their lives, characterized all members of the class. They demonstrated it by a proud identification as lawyers or teachers, by a determination to improve the contents of medicine or the procedures of a particular business, and by an eagerness to join others like themselves in a craft union, professional organization, trade association, or agricultural cooperative.[1]

The Blue Cross pioneers, many of them born in the years 1890 to 1910, along with their contemporaries in industry and the professions were a product of an optimistic period in American history that was expressed in the Blue Cross movement as in other aspects of American life.

The creation of multimillionaires and lesser millionaires and mass purchasing power coincided with the discovery and application of two specific medical developments which transformed the general hospital from a storehouse for the destitute to a healing institution for everyone, particularly those who could pay. These specific developments were antisepsis and anesthetics. The first made surgery relatively safe from postoperative infection, and the second made surgery relatively painless. Obviously, the rapidly emerging medical technology—and perhaps especially radiology, which spread rapidly after 1900—required capital to house the equipment and the patients. The prevailing philosophy of the role of government which limited it to police, post office, justice, sanitary environment, and universal education embodied no responsibility for personal health services except minimally for the destitute, transmitted from the Elizabethan poor laws through the English settlers in New England.

The American multimillionaires of the latter nineteenth and early twentieth centuries had little interest in individual poor people as a class—no Christmas baskets for selected, worthy poor families. They seemed rather to wish to use their surpluses, which accumulated rapidly and lavishly, for large scale community enterprises such as hospitals, libraries and colleges.

Consequently, the American hospitals were subsidized without interest or thought of repayment by the newly rich, and by contributions from the not-so-rich, in community after community across the nation. A few publicly financed general hospitals had been established for the poor in the larger cities. The mainstream of medical care in the United States became the voluntary hospital and the privately practicing physician who was able to make

---

[1] Robert H. Wiebe, *The Search for Order, 1877–1920* The Making of America Series (New York: Hill and Wang, 1967), p. 112.

arrangements with the hospital—first the surgeon and then the general practitioner and medical specialist for seriously ill medical patients, and still later the obstetricians and surgical specialists.[2] In exchange for the privilege of hospital appointments, the physicians were expected to provide care to indigent patients without charge. It is significant that private practice could be sustained by fees to private patients, with a politically tolerable residue of charity service. The voluntary hospital was tax exempt, chartered as a nonprofit institution, and therefore obliged to provide a modicum of free care. The charity tradition of hospitals has deep and old roots and persisted along after the general hospital became largely self-sustaining for day to day operating costs.

Thus the American health service delivery system became largely a private system both as to ownership of facilities and provisions of skills—the voluntary hospital and the physician in private practice. No other country has been able to support as expensive and as socially necessary a service by payments from a large middle income group, because the mass purchasing power was not present elsewhere. By 1920, the basic characteristics of the health service delivery system in the United States were stabilized. Until recently, the system has been largely provider-controlled, and the general public has been willing to accept and buy the services so organized and distributed; it is only recently that this provider-determined system has been encountering the forces of third party payment, government regulation, and direct consumer influence.

Between 1916 and 1918, attempts were made by 16 state legislatures from New York To California to establish some form of compulsory health insurance, essentially a mechanism to help families pay for health services, which were already being felt as costly and unpredictable episodes. The necessary mass political support in the states was not present, however, and the solid opposition of the American Medical Association, insurance companies, and the pharmaceutical industry, not to mention business and industry opposed to unaccustomed payroll taxes, stopped the movement. Its protagonists—leading intellectuals in labor economics, social work, medicine, and public health—had underestimated both the political appeal of universal health insurance and the strength of the opposition. The broad middle income group, the traditional and persistent political vital center, was not yet sufficiently aroused. The body politic was not yet prepared to think of health and welfare services in national terms until the depression produced the Social Security Act and established the framework for public policy regarding unemployment, pensions, and as a continuing subissue, the costly episodes of medical care.

[2]For a more extensive description of the development up to 1920, see Odin W. Anderson, *The Uneasy Equilibrium; Prive and Public Financing of Health Services in the United States 1875-1965* (New Haven, Connecticut: College and University Press, 1968).

It is possible, however, that there may be a relationship, if tenuous, between the Blue Cross developments in the 1930s and the hospital and medical care plans for lumberjacks in northern Wisconsin and the Pacific Northwest, railroad workers near isolated roundhouses throughout the West, and coal and iron miners in pits far from any amenities. Health services were made available to workers at these sites because they were remote from communities that could provide them. Emerging modern medicine, occupational hazards, and employer liability inspired these industrial health services for specific and isolated worker populations. Benefits for family members were not included. The few industrially based health services in populated areas evoked a great deal of attention among medical care reformers, but the concept did not spread far.

In the late 1920s and early 1930s, however, stimulated by the frequency and costliness of episodes of hospitalization, individual hospital prepayment plans appeared in Dallas, Texas, Grinnel, Iowa, Rockford, Illinois, and elsewhere. These single hospital plans appeared to be local responses to the wisdom of both stable financing for the hospital and prudent self-help for an occupational group with relatively low but steady income—teachers in the public schools, a group easy to organize and already accustomed to acting collectively.

The Dallas plan established at Baylor University Hospital by Justin F. Kimball, Ph.D., in 1929, was the one that received the greatest publicity.[3] Born in 1872, Kimball was a lawyer, educator, and administrator who had been superintendent of the Dallas public schools and subsequently became the executive vice-president of Baylor University. Several important elements converged in him: experience as a lawyer with insurance companies, knowledge of the financial problems of teachers (he doubled their salaries from 1914 to 1924), and experience with the teachers' sick benefit fund to replace income lost because of absence from work. Prepayment for hospital care was a natural extension. Undoubtedly, another important practical factor was Kimball's office manager, Bryce Twitty, to whom he could delegate administration of the hospital prepayment plan.[4] He worked from illness records of the sick benefit fund and the hospital records in Baylor University Hospital. Examining what he

---

[3] Data from a taped and transcribed interview with Dr. Justin F. Kimball by Melvin T. Munn on August 6, 1954, in Texas for the archives of the Blue Dross Commission on the occasion of the 25th anniversary of the Baylor plan. Kimball was 82 years of age at the time of the interview.

[4] From a taped and transcribed interview by Melvin T. Munn with Bryce Twitty in Tulsa, Oklahoma, on August 12, 1954, for the archives of the Blue Cross Commission. Twitty reports: ". . . it was sometime later (after Twitty's arrival) that Dr. Kimball and I were sitting in his office and I asked him why we couldn't do for sick people what lumber camps and railroads had done for their employees." Kimball said, " 'Good idea,' and he went to work with school teachers, and worked out a formula at 21 days." The plan grew sufficiently so as to require a full-time administrator.

could learn from the previous hospitalization experience of the teachers, Kimball calculated that the group as a whole had incurred an average of 15 cents a month in hospital bills. To assure a safe margin he established a rate of 50 cents a month, $6 a year per teacher, a modest figure even in 1929. Drawing on his community prestige, Kimball circulated all the school teachers in Dallas over his own signature, and 1,000 teachers were enrolled by the end of December, 1929, 75 percent of the group. Later, he enrolled the employees of the *Dallas News*; he knew the president of that newspaper well.[5]

It is significant that Kimball never conferred with the physicians associated with Baylor Hospital about the plan. "I carefully drew the plan so that it would not impinge or infringe in any way on a doctor's relationship between himself and his patient," he said. He was a good friend of Dr. E. H. Carey of Dallas, who later became the president of the AMA. Kimball apparently was not interested in expanding the hospital plan beyond its Baylor base. Even later, he paid no particular attention to Blue Cross development as such; he simply "spread the concept," as he put it. The value underpinning the voluntary movement was expressed in his own words: "I do think that the hospital plan rendered a service; it was a formula by which folks could help those who helped themselves."

The first time the experience of the Baylor plan was reported at an annual meeting of the American Hospital Association was in Toronto, Ontario, in 1931.[6] There was a request from AHA to have Kimball tell about the Baylor plan at that meeting. He was unable to be present but designated a substitute, who could not be found when the time came for his address. The chairman asked the audience if it would prefer to hear about "women's work" (hospital auxiliary) rather than the hospital prepayment plan. But the hospital plan prevailed, and Kimball's paper was read by the chairman, Asa Bacon, who later became one of the early supporters of Chicago's Blue Cross plan. Interestingly, two other Blue Cross pioneers, Frank Van Dyk and C. Rufus Rorem, who were also beginning to think about hospital prepayment, were at the AHA meeting but did not hear the Kimball paper.[7] Van Dyk had already been pondering the feasibility of some sort of prepayment plan in Essex County, New Jersey, and

[5]As an amusing sidelight. Frequently present in the small beginnings of a development, Twitty, Ibid, reported that only one person enrolled and the next day she had appendicitis. Soon 100 percent of the employees enrolled.

[6]Transactions of the 33rd Annual Convention of the American Hospital Association, Toronto, Ontario, September 28 to October 2, 1931, p. 669.

[7]Data from a taped and transcribed interview with Frank Van Dyk by Melvin T. Munn on July 23, 1954, in Chicago for the Blue Cross Commission in connection with the 25th anniversary of the Baylor plan. Data for Rorem from a taped and transcribed cassette of questions and answers that Rorem taped by himself following the writer's visit with him early in 1971.

Rorem reported that he was on the brink of a shift of interest from hospital accounting and capital investment to hospital prepayment.

The elements which converged to form the base for the Blue Cross development can be summarized:

1. A largely self-sustaining personal health services delivery system was capitalized by private philanthropy and community fund drives, with operating expenses for hospitals paid by private patients, and physicians in private practice who lived on fees to private patients.
2. Government had a minor role in personal health services, a problem to be handled on an individual basis along with food, clothing, shelter, and insurance against contingencies. The poor were provided health care by private charity and state and local governments. Health service for the poor was a residual of the prevailing voluntary system; a fringe of publicly supported general hospitals assisted in reducing the pressure of the poor on the voluntary system.
3. The concept of self-help through individual or group action in the private sector prevailed.
4. The general hospital became an increasingly costly service, so that even self-supporting families began to feel the impact of costly and unpredictable hospital care episodes.
5. A few single hospital prepayment plans began to appear providing leaven for spread of the prepayment concept.

From this base in the early thirties, prescient young men began to move. Within the American social, economic, and political context, the Blue Cross plans and subsequent prepayment and insurance developments were a natural and incremental response to family financial problems caused by the rapidly rising costs of personal health services. The Blue Cross idea was a group response to family financial problems without resort to government intervention. It was and is, within the American context, both an essentially conservative and innovative development, a feature which its early opponents did not understand. In fact, its promoters were sometimes called socialists! The Blue Cross promoters were steeped in the American dream of self-determination and private effort. Government was meant to govern, to provide a workable environment for private efforts, to set broad social goals, but to encourage the private sector to deliver the goods and services within certain legally established rules and regulations—a point still at issue.

The Populist and Progressive parties were then also in the American context essentially conservative movements to maintain democratic self-determination for open competition in the economy and direct access to the levels of political power—the first rural, based in the upper Middle West; and the second urban, based among intellectual social reformers. They were concerned mainly with the feared collusion of government and big business resulting in monopolies and high prices for railroad transport for crops and farm machinery. Another important concern was the felt unresponsiveness of elected officials to the ordinary citizen's needs and interests. The result was the institution of political devices such as referendum on public issues, recall of elected officials, and the direct primary.[8] Although there were no links between these political movements and the Blue Cross idea, they all believed in the values of self-help, self-determination, the balancing of the private and public sectors, and the diffusion of power in both sectors.

In interviews with the Blue Cross pioneers, I was struck with their complete acceptance of the premises of the American value system. Thus Blue Cross leaders had a philosophical consistency and an esprit de corps in the early days to sustain a relatively small group of men during many difficult times.

[8]See sources such as Benjamin Parke DeWitt, *The Progressive Movement; A Non-Partisian, Comprehensive Discussion of Current Tendencies in American Politics* (Seattle: University of Washington Press, 1968); Richard Hofstadter, *The Age of Reform from Bryan to FDR* (New York: Knopf, 1955); George E. Mowry, *The California Progressives* (Berkeley: University of California Press, 1951).

Chapter Four

Blue Cross and the American Political-Economic Model

The groundwork for the Blue Cross development was laid in a model of the liberal-democratic economic and political system which emerged during the nineteenth century and in which framework western countries try to cope with their public policy problems. Perhaps an explicit presentation of this model will help to clarify the economic and political context in which the Blue Cross idea developed and in which it continues to operate.

Central to the western economic and political model is the division of the economy into private and public sectors. The private sector was created by the middle class revolutions of the nineteenth century and resulted in the dismantling of the mercantile state. Suffrage eventually became universal regardless of class or sex. The principle became one person, one vote. Laws were enacted by legislators elected by the voters in open elections at regular intervals. A concept of checks and balances between the legislative, administrative, and executive branches of the government evolved, plus further checks and balances between the private and public sectors. This model is known as economic and political pluralism, the theory being that no one group at interest has enough power in relation to other groups to dominate, except temporarily. Its effective operation requires diversified interest groups who find it advantageous to engage in coalition politics, grouping and regrouping as the political issues change, a highly developed economy, and an informed electorate. Government becomes one of the large interest groups, which needs to be counterbalanced by the private sector. Even governments whose legislators are elected are not assumed necessarily to be custodians of the public interest; they might also reflect specific private interests. There is also a government apparatus called bureaucracy which tends to establish a life of its own.

Figure 4-1. Role of Government in the Private Sector

Market minimized			Market maximized	
		The electorate		
		The vital center of consensus among the electorate as to the private and public mix		
20%	30%		30%	20%
		Fundamental political values constant		

In this liberal-democratic model (shown in Figure 4-1) of an economic and political system, the political values are constant throughout the body politic—i.e., one person, one vote; representative government; government by explicit laws; an open system of freedom of speech, press, and assembly. But there are differing views among voters and interest groups as to the role of the government in influencing, controlling, or owning the means of production and distribution: For whose benefit? For what purpose? By what means of taxation?

The vital center of public consensus comprises approximately 60 percent of the electorate. Roughly 20 percent each are in the extreme "market minimized" and "market maximized" sectors. Politicians are usually unable to get elected unless they can draw votes from the left or right of the center line, extending far enough to include a few in the extreme left or right ends of the continuum. Conceivably, politicians can be elected solely within the vital center of 60 percent if the consensus is narrow enough to be contained completely within the vital center section. This is usually not the case. The tendency is to lean toward the market minimized end of the continuum or the market maximized end, depending on the mood of the electorate and the politicians as to the role of government in the means of production and distribution and the extent to which citizens can determine their own choices through the market rather than the ballot.[1]

---

[1] Recent sociological, economic, and political theorists who would support this model in principle and who are direct descendants of eighteenth century enlightenment political philosophies straight through the Federalist Papers and the American Constitution are: Robert A. Dahl, *Pluralistic Democracy in the United States—Conflict and Consent* (Chicago: Rand McNally, 1967); Robert A. Dahl and Charles E. Lindblom, *Politics, Economics and Welfare* (New York: Harper, 1953); Daniel J. Boorstin, *The Genius of American Politics* (Chicago: University of Chicago Press, 1953); Gerard DeGré, "Freedom and Social Structure," *American Sociological Review* 11 (October 1946) 529–536. Charles E. Lindblom, *The Intelligence of Democracy: Decision-Making Through Mutual Adjustment* (New York: Free Press, 1965); Walter Lippmann, *The Good Society: An Inquiry into the Principles of a Good Society* (New York: Little, Brown and Co., 1937); Arnold Rose, *The Power Structure: Political Process in American Society* (New York: Oxford, 1967);

It is evident that the more one belongs to the right extreme of the continuum (market +), the more one is likely to subscribe to limited government of the pre–World War I model and an open, competitive market economy on classical laissez faire lines. The more one belongs to the left extreme (market –), the more one is likely to favor public ownership of the means of production and distribution on classical socialistic lines, but within the political framework of representative government usually called democratic socialism. Naturally, one's place in the continuum will determine one's views toward the role of government in health and welfare policies, and also the form that health and welfare policies take.

As for welfare policies such as old age pensions, public assistance, and the so-called income maintenance programs, the premise of the right extreme (market +) is that citizens should arrange for their own old age, retirement, or disability, and their own personal health services. Tax funds are to be used for those who fall below certain minimums as determined by means tests. In substance, the individual is held accountable for his inability to earn his own way. On the left extreme (market –) the view is that government programs should cushion economic contingencies from the cradle to the grave. It is assumed that the individual is unable to cope with all the contingencies of life because of factors beyond his control. The ideal source of funding, according to this view, is the progressive income tax.

In western liberal democracies, what has resulted from the political debates over health and welfare measures and their financing has been a mix of means test, specified benefits for specified rights, payroll deductions, employer contributions, and progressive income tax. It was expected that an expanding social insurance program would eventually replace the means test–public assistance approach. The word "insurance" has been tenacious in the liberal-democratic social welfare lexicon. It implies the pooling of risk—as in life and fire insurance—by payments that are the same for everybody, given the same risks. It is steeped in the values of self-help, self-interest, foresight, contractual relationships, and paying your own way. It does not have any odor of income redistribution. Adding the warm word "social" gives the combined words "social insurance" an atmosphere both of togetherness and actuarial soundness.

Theodore Lowi, *The End of Liberalism: Ideology, Policy, and the Crisis of Public Authority* (New York: Norton, 1969); Milton Friedman, *Capitalism and Freedom* (Chicago: University of Chicago Press, 1963); Aaron Wildavsky, *The Politics of the Budgetary Process* (Boston: Little, Brown and Co., 1964); Harold L. Wilensky and Charles N. Lebeaux, *Industrial Society and Social Welfare* (New York: Russell Sage Foundation, 1958); James L. Sundquist, *Politics and Policy: The Eisenhower, Kennedy and Johnson Years* (Washington, D.C.: Brookings Institution, 1968).

The more one subscribes to the right side of the market $-$/market $+$ continuum, the more likely one is to favor privately owned insurance companies, and, further, profit-oriented insurance that covers risks such as fire, premature death, or high cost medical episodes. As one moves toward the far left of the continuum one eventually subscribes to a completely government-owned, government-financed, and salaried health service system financed by general tax revenues levied through a progressive personal and corporate income tax. On the right side, one is likely to favor cash indemnities for certain contingencies and financial controls such as deductibles and coinsurance. Providers of service are regarded as essentially autonomous units which the patient engages one by one or through a physician who is in effect a health service broker.

Toward the left extreme one moves through a variable mix of methods of delivering and financing health services toward the highly structured and completely financed government system. Services are "provided" rather than "purchased." There is no charge at time of service.

Critics of this pluralist economic model regard it as a caricature of the true state of affairs, because a large minority does not participate actively in interest group politics for reasons of ignorance, apathy, or inadequate resources. These shortcomings of the model are true and are a matter of degree; in all political systems so far derived, some groups have had a minimal share of power, for a host of reasons. The pluralist model, at least, keeps the options open and encourages participation, without the potential paternalism of the democratic socialist or welfare state models. The tension between individual autonomy and collective action threads through all of human history.

In general, the Blue Cross pioneers and current Blue Cross administrators range from just left of center to just short of the extreme right boundary of the vital center of the market continuum. This is an impression based on extensive interviews, writing, and public statements. It makes sense within the Blue Cross philosophy. The Blue Cross administrator reflects the essentially conservative character of the American electorate, who do not find sudden and drastic change congenial. Moreover, it seems likely that the positions in the market $-$/market $+$ spectrum of the members of the boards of directors of the Blue Cross plans over the country would be close to the positions of the plan administrators, on the assumption that congruence of views is necessary for workable relationships. Innovative plan administrators, however, need to help their boards face changing political realities effectively within the pluralist model presented.

Blue Cross leaders and administrators, past and present, are conservative but try to be innovative within the private sector. Whether they are

Figure 4–2. Position of Blue Cross Administrators on Market Continuum

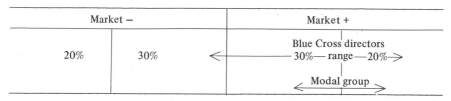

Market −				Market +
20%	30%		⟵───	Blue Cross directors ── 30%— range —20%—⟶ ⟵ Modal group ⟶

southern Democrats or northern Republicans, they regard themselves as political independents.[2] In keeping with their community roles, they try to maintain a low profile politically and a discreet but not necessarily complete detachment from partisan political activity. They try to maintain a fluid position between what Sundquist imaginatively describes as programmatic liberal Democrats or programmatic conservative Republicans,[3] i.e., those who are philosophically drawn to the respective extremes of the continuum, but maintain a dialogue with the moderates in the broad center.

[2]Two examples suffice and are selected because of their pithy replies to queries regarding their political inclinations: Frank Van Dyk, pioneer in the New Jersey and New York City Blue Cross plans, replied: "I have a hell of a time when I go to vote, because I don't vote along party lines," Frank Dickson of the Oregon plan said he was a Republican. The writer asked what this meant on the West Coast: "It means a little less liberal than the Democrats." From taped and transcribed interviews with Van Dyk in New York City on May 11, 1971, and with Dickson in Portland, Oregon, on April 30, 1972.

[3]James L. Sundquist, *Dynamics of the Party System: Alignment and Realignment of Political Parties in the United States* (Washington, D.C.: Brookings Institution, 1973), 239–240.

Chapter Five

Laying the Groundwork—The 1930s

During the late 1920s and early 1930s a man in Essex County, New Jersey, one in Chicago, one in St. Paul, and still another in Cleveland, unknown to each other and independently, were pondering the same possibility—some form of prepayment for families to pay for hospital care which would involve all the hospitals in the community. The man in New Jersey, son of a feed and grain dealer with only a grade school education, Frank Van Dyk, was a promoter-salesman. The man in Chicago, C. Rufus Rorem, son of a small town merchant in Iowa, was a certified public accountant with a Ph.D. in economics from the University of Chicago, a scholar and theorizer with a clear bent for systematic application. The man in St. Paul, E. A. van Steenwyk, son of a shoe and harness maker also from a small town in Iowa, with a two year teacher's certificate from Mankato State Teachers College in Minnesota and one year at the University of Minnesota, was a practical dreamer. John Mannix in Cleveland, son of an Irish immigrant family that experienced a great deal of illness in the twenties, had a high school education and was a self-taught hospital accountant with a flair for bold, large-scale action. The appropriate fusion of people with this variety of talents can result in a movement, and so it did.

At the beginning of the 1930s, Van Dyk was 33 years old, Rorem was 36, van Steenwyk 25, and Mannix 30. They embodied the old fashioned virtues of hard work, enlightened self-interest, enthusiasm, imagination, pragmatism, and dedication to the public interest. These characteristics were discernible in their writing and in interviews.[1] They were clearly products of a

---

[1] Van Steenwyk did not survive to be interviewed for this particular study but was well known to the author from the early forties to 1962, the year of his death. The author interviewed van Steenwyk's son John in Chicago on August 21, 1973, to gather personal history information.

stratum of American society trained from childhood to be self-reliant and to cope with facts, figures, and organizations. They were basically Calvinists, including the Roman Catholic Mannix and the Quaker Rorem.

Rorem was a graduate of Oberlin College (his Norwegian immigrant parents believed in education), and after graduate work at the University of Chicago he became an assistant professor of accounting in the business school there in 1928. That same year he met Michael M. Davis, over 15 years his senior, a Ph.D. in sociology from Columbia University in 1906, and for a long time a student of the economics of medical care and a crusader for health insurance. Davis was on the staff of the Julius Rosenwald Fund, a Chicago-based foundation established by Rosenwald of Sears, Roebuck & Co. to support activities that would help people to help themselves, as in grants for higher education of Negroes, for example. One of the interesting features of the fund was that it was to be in existence for 25 years, and thereafter liquidated and terminated. Rosenwald did not like self-perpetuating philanthropic foundations whose original objectives may become outmoded, and, in accordance with his stipulation, the fund was terminated in 1948.

Davis was in charge of a section on medical economics and was looking for a staff member who would do a study of capital investment in hospitals. Rorem became an associate on the staff. Davis was also active at the time in getting the Committee on Costs of Medical Care started. This was a research organization funded by six major foundations, Rosenwald among them, with a budget of $1 million, a large sum in those days for research in the economics of medical care. The Committee on the Costs of Medical Care published 26 reports on the incidence of illness, the use of and expenditures for personal health services, and group medical practice. The wide-ranging studies provided a factual base for personal health services for many years. They were a valiant attempt to introduce rationality into the emerging debates on health financing, voluntary and compulsory health insurance, and types of delivery systems.

Rorem said: "From my point of view we had picked the key point where all the conflicts and the changes were going to come."[2] He accepted Davis' offer to study capital investments in hospitals, a completely unexplored area. The study was sponsored by the Committee on the Costs of Medical Care. Rorem was then, in effect, a member of the staff of both the Rosenwald Fund and the CCMC. Beginning with the one on capital investment, a landmark study,[3] he carried out a series of investigations under CCMC's auspices.

[2]Interview with Rorem in New York City, December 17, 1970.
[3]C. Rufus Rorem, *The Public's Investment in Hospitals* (Chicago: University of Chicago Press, 1930).

Pursuing the nonprofit field further, the author asked Rorem if he did not like the profit field. *Rorem*: "I do not dislike the profit field. I was in business, as a salesman, for six years before entering college teaching. But public service was more attractive as a field of interest." *Anderson*: "Did you then have any feelings about the role of the nonprofit sector in the health field versus the government? Did you feel the nonprofit sector was a better method of funding health services than being dominated by the government?" *Rorem*: "I don't think I was conscious of that then." He felt that the private sector was good for experimentation. ... "Governments tend to emphasize equity, not efficiency; certainty, not originality. They do not provide the basis for much experiment or innovation, which are natural fields for private enterprise, whether nonprofit or commercial."

Rorem's original interest in capital investment in hospitals led quickly to interest in hospital prepayment. "The function of group hospitalization is not to make the problems of the hospital superintendent easier, but to solve the problems of the individual and of the public who own the hospitals," he said. "As long as hospital bills are unpredictable as to amount, people will complain about them. It is impossible to silence the popular criticism of hospitals by explaining that hospitals are efficiently managed or that hospital bills are reasonable." These are two separate, though interrelated, problems, a persistent concern of Blue Cross plans to this day: Do they represent the public or the hospitals? Does it make any difference? Many attempts at resolving these questions will be revealed as the Blue Cross story unfolds.

Rorem's connection with the American Hospital Association was established as a member and sometime chairman of its Committee on Uniform Hospital Accounting from 1931 to 1936. Serious discussion on hospital prepayment at annual meetings of AHA began in 1932. In 1933, AHA formed a special group known as the Council on Community Relations and Administrative Practice. Rorem became this council's part-time consultant on group hospitalization, but with his office still at the Rosenwald Fund on Chicago's south side, and on the fund's payroll.

Early in 1933, Rorem gave his first full-scale presentation, as reported by him, on "what the periodic payment plan for the purchase of hospital care has thus far demonstrated," mainly a paper on the principles and theory of prepayment, and also in 1933, Rorem published his first article on group hospitalization in *Modern Hospital*. He was beginning to write on the subject even before concrete experience of any magnitude was available for investigation. During the thirties, hospital prepayment plans surfaced in Essex County, New Jersey; St. Paul, Minnesota; Charleston and Bluefield, West Virginia, and Sacramento, California. Rorem drew a great deal of his background material from the CCMC studies; by 1936, he had published 43 articles on hospital prepayment and a range of other related subjects, beginning to draw on actual experience.[4]

From 1934 to 1936 Rorem spent almost all his time in the promotion and development of hospital prepayment, making trips to all parts of the United States to consult with communities contemplating such plans. In due course, he became acquainted with Van Dyk in New Jersey and van Steenwyk in St. Paul.

Rorem and John Mannix were concurrent in their interests in group hospitalization, though it may be that Mannix' interest preceded Rorem's. Both became recognized consultants in group hospitalization development shortly after the American Hospital Association endorsed the principle of prepayment in 1933. Both men also had an early interest in hospital finance and accounting which eventually, and perhaps logically, led to an interest in group hospitalization.

In 1921, at the age of 21, Mannix took a position in the accounting department of Mt. Sinai Hospital in Cleveland. His office was close to the cashier's and he had an opportunity to watch the reactions of patients to their hospital bills. He observed that they usually reacted to small, itemized charges rather than the total bill, and it occurred to him that an average daily charge would be logical and would help to allay, at least in part, patient dissatisfaction with hospital bills.[5]

In 1926 Mannix became administrator of the Elyria Memorial Hospital in Elyria, Ohio, where he established inclusive hospital rates for tonsillectomies and maternity cases on an average derived from examination of the billings of many patients. In 1927, it occurred to him that "I could take the total charges for room service and extras and divide these not only among people hospitalized but among all people, whether they were hospitalized or not, and have everybody pay. This was a brand new idea to me, and only to me. Then I found out that the same principle had been used many times before in other areas." He induced a local insurance company to issue a contract for hospital service in Elyria in 1928–29, but it was not a success. Mannix said: "I think many people who were involved in the early Blue Cross program, all of whom started pretty independently, all thought they had original ideas."

In 1930 he joined the administrative staff of the Western Reserve University medical complex in Cleveland, where he remained for nine years. This

---

[4]In a letter to the author, May 20, 1971, he wrote impishly that when he first became interested in hospital prepayment he scoured the library for literature on the subject. Finding none, he concluded that if he wanted something to read he would have to write it himself.

[5]Interview in Cleveland, February 24, 1971.

gave him a much stronger base from which to promote group hospitalization. While at University Hospital he consulted in the development of Blue Cross plans in Cleveland and Detroit. The Michigan consultation had significance for the future, as he became the first Blue Cross administrator there in 1939.

Mannix met Rorem while they were both members of the Committee on Hospital Accounting of the American Hospital Association. They had a mutual interest in hospital accounting and also in some new method of financing hospital care for the public. Mannix reported that during the late 1930s "Rufus [Rorem] and I were always very cooperative in all this—helping plans to get started. There was never the slightest competition between us. As a matter of fact, at that point people were getting help wherever they could find it." Under the circumstances, competition was hardly necessary.

Consultations by Mannix and Rorem were going on at about the same time bellwether hospital plans were being established in Newark, New Jersey, and St. Paul, Minnesota, under the leadership of Frank Van Dyk and E. A. van Steenwyk, respectively. The Essex County (New Jersey) plan in 1933, preceded the one in St. Paul by a margin of only six months. Mannix and Rorem, among others, give credit to Van Dyk for starting the first multihospital prepayment plan, a concept central to both Mannix and Rorem in their consultations. Three other plans were started in 1933—in Charleston and Bluefield, West Virginia and San Jose, California.[6]

As it turned out, Van Dyk and van Steenwyk were the first organizers and operators of what became major Blue Cross plans. Van Dyk had been among other things on a newspaper in Paterson, New Jersey, for two years, in public relations and advertising. Then from 1922 to 1931, he was on the staff of a hospital fundraising concern in New York. In 1930 he was commissioned to make a hospital survey in Essex County, New Jersey, and during that year he also conducted four hospital fund drives in various parts of the country. They all were successful, but the stock market crash of 1929 eventually overtook the fundraising firm, and he was out of a job. He recovered quickly and became the first director of the newly created Hospital Council in Newark in February 1931.

One function Van Dyk had as director of the Hospital Council was to collect overdue hospital accounts for the 14 hospitals in Newark and Essex County. This was a trying experience. As Van Dyk reported: ". . . it occurred to me what a wonderful thing it would be if you could remove the cashier's window from the hospital." Asking people to pay $2 on a hospital bill during

---

[6]Technically, the first multihospital plan (two hospitals) was established in Sacramento, California, in 1932. It was first known as the Superior California Hospital Plan and later as the Inter-Coast Hospitalization Association. It was quite limited in scope and operation. In the late 1940s, it was dropped from the Blue Cross approval list because it delegated enrollment to an outside agency.

the depression was "such a tragic thing. There ought to be a better method of doing things."[7]

Like Rorem, Van Dyk looked for literature on hospital insurance. This was at the time of the emerging reports of the CCMC, which he read. He said the reports "hinted about the prepayment idea. So all these thoughts were running in my mind, and then I remembered hearing something about this idea . . . at some hospital convention."[8]

Van Dyk reported that in 1932 two men from Texas visited Newark promoting the idea of selling insurance for hospitals on a commission basis, but "these people were interested only in making money." A prominent local real estate dealer, Louis Schlesinger, was also visited by these promoters. Schlesinger suggested that he and Van Dyk go to Dallas and talk with the people in the Baylor plan.

So, in 1932, Van Dyk and the real estate sponsor went to Dallas. Van Dyk visited with Kimball and Twitty. He was looking for actuarial data and was greatly disappointed that there were none. He wanted to know about charges, margins, and reserves. "They didn't know anything about that. They just collected the money. It was more money than they had before, so what the hell. That was their philosophy at the time. There were no records as to incidence." Van Dyk came home from Texas convinced of two things: He learned from one physician that there needed to be free choice of hospital in a community, and some actuarial data, however, crude, were needed to estimate costs. Two other hospitals in Dallas had parallel group hospital plans, and Van Dyk also felt that three single hospital plans in one community were confusing and divisive.

On returning to Newark, Van Dyk gathered data on use of hospital care in a presumably average employed group in Essex County, where he was still executive secretary of the Hospital Council. Also using CCMC data, he estimated that 7 percent of the members of the employed group received hospital care in a year, for an average length of stay of 10 days. Assuming 30,000 members, with 7 percent admitted to hospitals during a year, the resulting 2,100 patients would use 21,000 days of hospital care a year. He learned that Baylor had also averaged 10 days, "so let us be conservative and figure 11 days. The total number of days of 30,000 members would then be 23,100. Since we estimated income would be $180,000, at $6 per member per

---

[7]Interview in New York City, May 11, 1971. Also interview conducted by Melvin Munn for Blue Cross Commission in connection with the 25th anniversary of the Baylor plan, Chicago, July 23, 1954.

[8]American Hospital Association, Toronto, Ontario, 1931.

year, we had a per diem of $7.80."[9] In those days, that was enough to reimburse the hospitals and pay expenses.

Van Dyk wrote up his actuarial calculations in an article published by the American Hospital Association in January 1933. He referred to it as his "17 page report" and was proud of it because according to him it was the first attempt to estimate hospital use for hospital prepayment purposes.[10]

Concurrently, the CCMC studies were yielding data on hospital use by a representative sample of the population. I. S. Falk, then a staff member of CCMC, reported that in 1933 he was approached by Louis Dublin and Lee Frankel, statisticians for Metropolitan Life Insurance Co., about estimates for hospital admissions and length of stay. This was Falk's first contact with the hospital prepayment development. He said: "I can still remember saying to Louis [Dublin] 'That is very easy to do.' A quick look at the available data showed about one day of hospital care per capita per annum. I said to him, 'The available data indicate that a day of hospital care on the average costs about so much. So add 10 or 15 percent to that figure, and that is your premium. It is as simple as that.' "[11] Although Van Dyk was aware of the CCMC data, he preferred data from the area where he was interested in starting a hospital prepayment plan. His estimates were lower than those of CCMC.

The fourth man who can be identified as a Blue Cross pioneer is E. A. van Steenwyk, who had already had a risk-taking career before he was 30 years old. The stock market crash of 1929 broke an apparently successful venture in residential real estate in Chicago.[12] Before 1929, van Steenwyk had taught school for a year, then went to the University of Minnesota, where he was active in drama. He had also attempted to start a literary magazine. After the abortive business venture in Chicago, he and his wife left for southern Minnesota with an old car and $40 in cash—their only possessions. In Minnesota, they lived in an old log cabin on his wife's family farm.

Van Steenwyk became acquainted with the hospital field by selling advertising in the journal *Minnesota Hospital*, in addition to the *Minnesota Horticulturist*. In order to sell advertising in a hospital journal effectively, he tried to learn about hospitals and their characteristics. He quit when he was

[9]Frank Van Dyk, "A Group Hospital Insurance Plan," *Bulletin of the American Hospital Association* 7 (January 1933) 45–60.

[10]Interview, May 11, 1971.

[11]Interview in New Haven, Connecticut, April 2, 1971.

[12]Interview with his son John in Chicago, August 21, 1973, and interview by Melvin Munn in Philadelphia on July 28, 1954, for the Blue Cross Commission in connection with the 25th anniversary of the Baylor plan. Van Steenwyk died in 1962 at the age of 57.

offered a salary, after having worked on a commission. Through his hospital advertising experience, however, he got to know two leading hospital superintendents in St. Paul, Peter Ward, M.D. and Arthur M. Calvin. They had learned about the Baylor plan at the New Orleans meeting of the American Hospital Association in 1932 and were interested in starting such a plan in St. Paul. Discussions between Ward, Calvin, and van Steenwyk late in 1932 resulted in creation of the second multihospital prepayment plan, and van Steenwyk became its director in March 1933. Enrollment started in July. Van Steenwyk had been exposed to the CCMC reports; he knew something about the Essex County development and met Van Dyk in 1933. He was then 28 years old.

In the pattern of the early years, van Steenwyk was a one man show until there was some growth. He did everything: management, enrollment, hospital relations, and promotion—including radio advertising. A favorite story of his was that after making a spot announcement at the radio station about the availability of group hospitalization and his plan, he had to sprint back to his office a few blocks away to take telephone calls, because there was no one else there.

One of van Steenwyk's contributions was creation of the Blue Cross symbol. He had a flair for communication and enlisted a poster artist in his search for an attractive and simple symbol. The first symbol was a picture of a nurse in a blue and white uniform, which was used in Minnesota and elsewhere for some years but never really caught on.[13] The symbol that did take hold was a blue cross with short bars of equal length and width. In 1934 the name Blue Cross and the symbol were first used to identify nonprofit hospital plans, starting with van Steenwyk's St. Paul plan. In 1941, when Blue Cross plans became eligible for institutional membership in the American Hospital Association, the member plans were permitted to identify themselves by using the seal of AHA superimposed on a blue cross as a legally protected mark.

By the end of 1935, 15 plans had been established in 11 states, and during 1936 six more plans were initiated. Concurrently, there was a move to create a coordinating agency of some sort to give the now rapidly growing movement a national focus and a broad base. Frank Van Dyk, who had moved from Essex County to start the plan in New York City in 1935, gave Rufus Rorem credit for moving the emerging plans to think in terms of a national organization and a national system.

According to Rorem, the Rosenwald Fund had decided to terminate its Division of Medical Economics partly because it had become too contro-

---

[13] Interviews with Abbott Fletchei, long-time board member of Minneapolis-St. Paul Blue Cross and its general counsel, Minneapolis, August 12, 1972; and Bert O'Leary, long-time employee hired by van Steenwyk in St. Paul, August 12, 1972.

versial.[14] There were long-time personal relationships involved. Davis had known Julius Rosenwald since 1915, and became a personal friend of Lessing Rosenwald, his son.[15] The settlement that was made with the officers of the fund in 1936 (the elder Rosenwald had died in 1932), was a clear example of venture capital from philanthropic foundations in the best American tradition.

Davis and Rorem were each given custody over a substantial amount of money for those days, $175,000 and $100,000 respectively, for four years. Rorem later received an extension of one year and an additional $25,000. The conditions were that the money should be spent in the field of medical economics and that a nonprofit agency or agencies be found to which the fund could legally grant money. Davis set up his own agency, known as the Committee for Research in Medical Economics, which was concerned with research and promotion of national health insurance. Although Davis' interests were broad in the medical care field, his public image was clearly associated with the heated controversy over national health insurance. His agency also established the first journal of research in the economics of medical care, known as *Medical Care*.

Rorem took the voluntary, nonprofit route and sought an agency through which he could promote group hospitalization and uniform accounting as a tool of administration. Rorem and Davis were not necessarily at odds regarding the future sponsorship of health insurance in the United States. They sought each other's counsel frequently after they separated in 1936. Davis saw voluntary health insurance as a stage leading to some form of national health insurance, and to that degree was sympathetic and pragmatic.[16]

Rorem, on the other hand, was willing to give the private, nonprofit sector a good try, hoping it would succeed. He had no particular aversion, however, to health insurance becoming a government program. Pressed on this point in our interview, Rorem said: "In the field at the time I was thought of as a safe man. Mike Davis was considered dangerous by organized medicine. As a matter of fact, I was probably more radical in many respects. I never believed that private practice and commercial insurance could solve the problems of providing and financing health service. It seemed to me that they were important parts of the problem." It is difficult to determine how Rorem's attitude affected his relationships in the field, but undoubtedly it must have done so.[17] In the

[14] Interview, December 17, 1970.

[15] Interview with Michael Davis in Chevy Chase, Maryland, February 7, 1971. Dr. Davis died in 1972.

[16] Interview, February 7, 1971.

[17] *Anderson*: "Really, you were less doctrinaire than Davis was." *Rorem*: "That is one of the reasons I never had a heart attack. I tried to keep the areas in which I got excited under control. But I had plenty of excitement, and there was a continuous struggle for power." Interview, December 17, 1970.

market +/market — continuum, Rorem might be placed left of center ideologically and right of center operationally; he played the whole range within the extremes. This may be one of the reasons he did not go to the American Hospital Association first with his Rosenwald Fund nest egg during a depressed economic period. From the start, Rorem regarded group hospitalization as the public's plan and not that of the hospitals, and therefore he preferred to find an agency that did not represent hospitals.

He went first to the Twentieth Century Fund, but somebody there was already working in medical economics and did not want competition. The next choice was the Community Chest and Councils of America. The chest was sympathetic but turned the offer down because group hospitalization was not concerned with charity but with self-supporting people. The third choice, which ended the search, was the American Hospital Association. Robin Buerki, M.D., who was then AHA president, was at that time director of hospitals at the University of Wisconsin. Rorem reported that the association officers who considered his proposal "had a quick meeting, and they grabbed it immediately. Even though they were some of the most conservative people, they saw a chance to get going." Aside from personalities, there may have been an understandable caution on the part of the American Hospital Association. The only professional member of the staff was Bert W. Caldwell, M.D., the executive secretary, and according to Rorem he was apprehensive about such an independent project. The Rev. Maurice F. Griffin, a trustee of AHA and a close friend of Caldwell, assured him that the venture would be a good thing. As Rorem put it, the only two males at AHA headquarters were Caldwell and the janitor. When Rorem arrived there was a third. Rorem was given the title of associate secretary of the association. AHA was a struggling organization at that time, and recognition by a well-known philanthropic foundation was salutary.

A body known as the Committee on Hospital Service was created, but AHA was not corporately represented on it. According to Rorem, the only thing Caldwell was asked to do as executive secretary was to sign checks: "We were a de facto self-determining organization. We would report to the trustees when we thought there was something interesting to report, not because we thought it was any of their business."

Rorem naturally had a great deal to do with appointment of the initial members of the Committee on Hospital Service. He remarked that it never occurred to him to ask any of the people administering plans to be on the first committee, nor for that matter any hospital men as such: "The venture seemed to me to be essentially a public affair, and each member of the first committee had a record of public awareness; they could be relied on to keep hospital influence in its proper bounds."[18]

In Addition to Rorem as secretary, the following people were members of the first committee for a five year term beginning in the autumn of 1936:

- Basil C. MacLean, M.D. (41), administrator, Strong Memorial Hospital, Rochester, N.Y., chairman; AHA president, 1942, after he went off the committee. He was a personal friend of Rorem. Protestant. Rorem, then 42, was a Quaker.
- Robin C. Buerki, M.D. (44), administrator, Wisconsin General Hospital; AHA president when the committee was formed.
- Sigismund S. Goldwater, M.D. (62), commissioner of hospitals, New York City; hospital consultant; former administrator, Mt. Sinai Hospital, New York City; AHA president, 1908. A leading figure for the Jewish constituency.
- Rev. Maurice F. Griffin (54), AHA trustee; Catholic Hospital Association officer; AHA distinguished service award (1944); later a monsignor. A leading figure for the Catholic constituency.

To bring in the hospital plans, Rorem early in 1937 arranged for an advisory group of hospital plan executives, which in 1938 became the Council on Hospital Service Plans of the American Hospital Association. In 1939, the council was enlarged to include a few hospital administrators.

By 1941 the grant from the Rosenwald Fund, including the one year extension of the original four year term, was terminating, and the Committee on Hospital Service had to look around for other means of support in order to sustain itself as a national agency for the local Blue Cross plans. It was decided that the national federation of plans would be supported by dues from the member plans in the form of institutional membership in the American Hospital Association. In 1941, the name was changed to the Hospital Service Plan Commission. The commission was a separate financial entity but operated within the AHA corporate structure. The two agencies were now in a much closer working relationship.

Rorem related that a central and protracted problem while he was in the committee and the commission office (1936–1946) was clarification of the relationship between a Blue Cross plan and its contracting hospitals. There were

[18]Personal communication, August 1, 1973.

two conflicting points of view: (1) that Blue Cross was a conduit for money going to hospitals, which were the parent or senior sponsoring agencies, and (2) that Blue Cross was essentially a public service agency responsible to its enrollees and the total public.[19] There was no unanimity within the commission membership on this question, nor was there a prevailing view among the executives of the burgeoning hospital plans.

As national coordinator, Rorem tried valiantly to solidify Blue Cross philosophy and principles—with apparent success on the surface but with constant restiveness underneath. In 1938 the Committee on Hospital Service had adopted a now classic set of principles for approval of plans, as follows:

1. They were incorporated as nonprofit organizations and therefore had no stockholders, investments, or profits for individuals.
2. Their boards of directors represented hospitals, physicians, and the general public.
3. They were supervised by state insurance or other appropriate departments.
4. As nonprofit corporations they held low cash reserves, since hospitals were to provide a reserve of service instead of cash.
5. They placed emphasis on hospital benefits in the form of service rather than cash indemnities.
6. The established plans were not in competition with other plans.
7. They placed all employees on salaries and offered no commissions to salesmen.

From 1933 to the time these principles were adopted the emerging hospital plans were operating on implicit principles such as nonprofit multihospital, and service benefit. It was out of this welter of implicit principles that Rorem tried to bring some order. As reported by J. Douglas Colman: "One of the many things I give Rufus Rorem great credit for is that he encouraged all of us to get enabling legislation and lay the basic groundwork that this was a community service agency. He laid down the principles on which we operated, and gave them visibility, gave them credibility, gave them integrity. It just never would have had the national unity, diverse as it is, had it not been for Rufus."[20] Even so, Rorem remarked that the idea of Blue Cross as a form of social insurance was not widely accepted by the hospital field, nor by many of the promoters and developers of the Blue Cross movement.[21]

[19] Ibid.

[20] A Blue Cross pioneer who was with Van Dyk in New Jersey and later became director of Maryland Blue Cross and, still later, Associated Hospital Service, the Blue Cross plan of New York City, interview in New York City, January 9, 1971.

[21] Question and answer tape made by Rorem for this book early in 1971.

The importance of enabling legislation to the Blue Cross development can hardly be exaggerated. Very early, Blue Cross plans needed to be differentiated from private insurance companies. It was advantageous and logical to seek nonprofit status and not be subject to the usual insurance laws requiring large cash reserves and taxes on surpluses. State after state passed enabling legislation as a response to the need for a form of insurance that legislators felt it was expedient to exclude from the regular insurance laws. Rorem formulated a model law for the states to adopt.[22]

By 1940 there were 39 plans in operation with a total enrollment of over four million. There were 17 plans in the East, seven in the South, 11 in the Middle West, and four in the West (two on the West Coast). Blue Cross concentrations were in the East, more specifically in New York City, Boston, Philadelphia; in the Middle West in Cleveland, Detroit, Chicago, and the Twin Cities; in the South in New Orleans; and in Denver in the West. Each plan had started on a shoestring with various sources of funding: foundation grants, community chest grants, loans, hospital contributions. The start-up budgets were rarely projected for longer than three months; then they had to generate income to pay operating costs. Frequently hospitals would provide back-up service without charge until the plan was operating in the black. Without exception, as far as I could determine, all start-up money and hospital deficits were eventually paid back by the plans.

Even though Rorem felt that the general commitment to the Blue Cross idea as a community service and in a social insurance context was not uniform across the country, the leadership in the emerging centers of power certainly subscribed to his principles and gave the movement the essential image that Rorem and others desired.[23] Obviously, the Blue Cross concept was struggling with ambiguities in the American value system itself: the balance between nonprofit and profit enterprises in the provision of goods and services, not to mention the balance between the private and public sectors.

Even in the 1930s personal health services were already a big business as measured in dollars; over $3 billion a year, 4 percent of the gross national product, was spent for health services. Total expenditures for hospital care were pushing toward $1 billion; estimated investments in hospitals totaled between $3.5 and $4 billion. There were close to 400,000 beds in nonfederal

[22] Odin W. Anderson, *State Enabling Legislation for Non-Profit Hospital and Medical Plans, 1944*, School of Public Health, Public Health Economics, Research Series No. 1 (Ann Arbor: University of Michigan, 1944).

[23] There is no doubt that there was general enthusiasm among plan directors. Harold Maybee, who started the Delaware plan in 1935 at the age of 30, said in an interview in Wilmington, Delaware, on November 14, 1972: "In the early days we did everything but sweep out the office. We were positively messianic in our ardor. We believed. We were all involved with it. There were some who went along for the ride. But in general the early

short-term general and special hospitals.[24] The funds provided for start-up costs for hospital prepayment were modest, given this financial base, but an important factor was the promise of participating hospitals to provide service for a limited period without charge until revenue started to come in. In any case, it would seem that the hospital industry had a large enough "critical mass" to back a movement whose future was uncertain. The risk for the hospitals was minimal. The risk for the plan directors was maximal—their jobs.

The hospitals and community leaders responded to the hospital prepayment idea intuitively within the American value system and with American entrepreneurial know-how that was missing in other western countries, with the exception of Canada, where voluntary prepayment eventually was phased out when that country embarked on national health insurance. The board members of voluntary hospitals had, and have, a predominant represen-tation of business leadership. Hospital administrators were, and are, accustomed to operating in financial and managerial terms. Adding a new financing mechanism for the self-sustaining element of the population was, in the context, a natural and congenial development. This is not to say that the Blue Cross idea started out as naturally and simply as this brief summary may imply. Few people think theoretically about a new social invention or development. Even Rorem, the foremost theoretician of them all, said what he proposed seemed so natural and reasonable that it was hardly debatable—self-help, community orientation, and nonprofit because money should not be made at the expense of sick people. The statistical underpinning giving the movement some operating predictability was the uneven cost of hospitalized illness for a family in a year—in short, insurance, but insurance with a difference.[25]

The drive and enthusiasm for the Blue Cross idea originated with the early pioneers, not the hospitals. Hospitals were timid in their backing of prepayment in the 1930s. Describing one locality but generalizing to others, Colman reported that the hospitals in Essex County, New Jersey, hoped the prepayment plan would be successful enough to pay dues to the Hospital

---

leaders were all just bubbling over with ideas. We'd get together, and bull sessions would last until two, three o'clock in the morning. I don't think money was the prime incentive. They were enchanted with the idea. They were enthusiastic like a scientist who wanted to make a breakthrough into something, and . . . you have a good taste left in your mouth."

[24] Data from Monroe Lerner and Odin W. Anderson, *Health Progress in the United States: 1900-1960*, Chapters 22 and 23 (Chicago: University of Chicago Press, 1963), pp. 229-245.

[25] Mannix, for example, said in an interview in Cleveland on February 24, 1971: "We [the early Blue Cross leaders] just took it for granted that you wouldn't do it any other way."

Council and that the work the council was doing could be financed as a by-product of the prepayment plan: "All this notion that it was going to solve the financial problems of hospitals was farthest from their minds. Nobody dreamed it was going to grow to the size that it did."[26]

In retrospect, the number of developments from 1933 to 1940 seems incredible. The early Blue Cross executives were men facing many unknowns. Originally, the plans covered only employees and not their dependents; the dependents were an unknown and feared quantity actuarially. But common sense and equity would shortly have it that dependents should be covered too, and so they were. Another issue was the inclusion of maternity benefits. Maternity was assumed to be an uninsurable risk because it was "premeditated." Nevertheless, maternity benefits became a standard part of the family service package.

From the beginning the method of paying hospitals was of crucial importance in plan-hospital relationships, intensified as hospital income came increasingly from the plans. In general, plans started to pay the same rates to all hospitals, negotiated on a per diem basis. Then the method of payment shifted to a sliding scale depending on the length of stay, the first few days being allowed a higher rate, although the rates were still uniform for all hospitals. The uniform rate for all hospitals was obviously untenable, given the great differences among hospitals in size, services, proportion of charity patients, and medical teaching affiliations, to mention a few of many factors. So the next stage was one of varying rates for different hospitals, related in some way to their costs or charges.

The entrance of large third party payers on a contract basis necessitated some kind of national rate structure more or less satisfactory to both the providers and the payers. An important force moving in the direction of uniformity in reimbursement policy, in addition to the Blue Cross plans, was the Emergency Maternity and Infant Care program (EMIC) administered by the U.S. Children's Bureau, through the state health departments, for the wives and dependents of men in the military service during World War II. This was the first nationwide, uniform program paying for health care for a segment of the population using the voluntary hospital, private practice system. Although limited to the wives and dependents of men in service, the program was of sufficient magnitude to contribute significantly toward the rationalization of hospital rates paid by third parties. The program was in operation from early 1943 to late 1946. During that period approximately 1,164,000 maternity cases

[26]Interview, January 9, 1971.

and 190,000 infant care cases were paid for.[27] The EMIC program provided detailed procedures for determining cost; the American Hospital Association provided a cost accounting manual. In so far as possible, the federal government, through the Children's Bureau, had to know what it was buying. Hospitals were entering a period of cost accountability which theretofore had not been required of them. Private patients had always paid hospitals as billed; philanthropy and state public welfare departments paid according to custom, usually less than what was billed to private patients, and deficit financing of some sort made up the difference. Large third party contractual buyers led to detailed scrutiny of cost allocations that were never considered by individual private patients. In time, but a long time given the importance and magnitude of hospital financing, increasingly sophisticated costing and reimbursement methods were devised.

In the early Blue Cross days deduction from employees' pay checks by the employer was an innovation which most employers were reluctant to undertake. Instead, the plans designated an employee in each group, or the employees chose one, to collect subscription or membership payments periodically from other employees. Gradually employers began to provide the important service of payroll deduction. The passage of the Social Security Act in 1936, which stipulated payroll deductions for the federal retirement benefit program, had set a legal precedent for payroll deductions, and labor union —management negotiations to include payroll deduction of union dues had made headway by 1940.

In the early days the same subscription rate was charged all employed groups in a Blue Cross plan's jurisdiction regardless of age and sex composition and occupation, although the rates were different for family and single contracts, and for ward or semiprivate service. The method of charging all groups the same rates became known as "community rating." The method known as "merit or experience rating," in which rates are established according to the cost experience of a particular group, has a long history among private insurance companies. Group hospitalization experience usually varies according to the age, sex, and occupational composition of a covered employed group. Blue Cross plans initially had adopted the community rate method, which was simple to administer and equitable, given the community orientation of Blue Cross plans. In time the community rating versus experience rating issue became a soul-searching one for Blue Cross administrators as competition from private insurance companies intensified.

[27]Nathan Sinai and Odin W. Anderson, *E.M.I.C.; A Study of Administrative Experience,* School of Public Health, Bureau of Public Health Economics, Research Series No. 3 (Ann Arbor: University of Michigan, 1948).

Chapter Six

Achieving a Base—The 1940s

At the beginning of 1940, Blue Cross had attained a nationwide enrollment of around six million members in 56 plans. By 1945, the enrollment was up to 19 million in 80 plans, and by the early 1950s it was 40 million. By that time, private insurance companies were also coming up from behind, after an early lack of interest in insuring against hospital costs.

In addition to an intense public interest in some form of insurance against hospital costs and physician costs, there were important external factors which had a direct effect on the accelerated growth. McIntyre calls the period of the 1940s and early 1950s the "years of the fringes,"[1] It was a time of rapid increases in personal income taxes, stimulating interest in fringe benefits as a form of tax reduction. The taxes on profits of corporations were increased, and the rules governing the taxability of employer contributions to pension and profit-sharing plans were made more liberal. In 1942, the National War Labor Board approved wage increases in the form of nonwage benefits. In 1947 and 1949, the National Labor Relations Board and the U.S. Supreme Court ruled that employer contributions to insurance, including health insurance, and pension plans were "wages" and therefore could be included in collective bargaining. Accordingly, fringe benefits became an increasingly important element in employer personnel policies. All these developments were incentives for enrollment in hospital and medical insurance and prepayment plans.

At the same time, Blue Cross plans were facing several major problems. Perhaps the most important was the increasing restiveness of hospitals with the contractual relationship guaranteeing service at a negotiated price.

[1]Duncan M. McIntyre. *Voluntary Health Insurance and Rate Making*. Ithaca (New York: Cornell University Press, 1962), p. 146.

45

George Bugbee, for example, executive director of the American Hospital Association from 1943 to 1954, was ever watchful of Blue Cross reimbursement amounts and methods. He regarded his role as chiefly one of looking after the financial interests of hospital, and of AHA constituents, and establishing a strong hospital service base for the public. He saw Blue Cross plans as merely one of several sources of hospital income. In fact, he felt that "Blue Cross had outbargained the hospitals."[2]

Another problem was the need to have some sort of package benefit plan which included physicians' services and hospital services, at least surgical services in the hospital, and perhaps also other physicians' services. Physicians' services were also regarded now as an insurable risk, particularly surgery. Still another problem was the need for the hospital plans to cooperate with one another in enrolling national accounts of employers with employees in several states, such as the steel, automobile, and food processing industries. Some large private insurance companies were already geared to national accounts because they could sell health insurance in all states. Insurance companies had the added attractiveness to employers of selling a one-package service: life and disability insurance, pensions, and personal health services. Blue Cross plans had discovered that members traveled and found themselves needing hospital care outside the jurisdictions of their home plans. Some means of arranging for service under these circumstances was obviously called for. Also, there was a need for a mechanism by which Blue Cross members who moved to an area with another Blue Cross plan could transfer their memberships without repeating the exclusions and waiting periods to which they were subject on their initial enrollment. No such problem existed for insurance comapnies since they could sell insurance nationally and paid cash indemnities, not services delivered by contracting hospitals. Finally, there was the threat to voluntary health insurance that the Congress might enact some form of universal health insurance legislation—a threat that was constantly simmering on the back burner of the congressional kitchen stove, beginning in the late 1930s and continuing until President Truman left office.

These problems seemed to occur all at once. Undoubtedly, leaders in the field were worrying about all of them simultaneously, and it may have been the easiest one that was tackled first. Stuart[3] and Van Dyk were among the leaders who proposed in 1943 that all the plans join in reciprocal arrangements to provide benefits for members of any plan hospitalized away from home, to

---

[2]Interview, Genesee Depot, Wisconsin, March 17, 1971.
[3]James E. Stuart, director of Cincinnati Blue Cross and, later, First president of the Blue Cross Association.

allow free transfer of membership between plans, and to help in enrolling any national account that involved several plans. The one page document that emerged through the Hospital Service Plan Commission in 1944 became an article of faith, but it lacked details about how to make the arrangement work. Serious administrative difficulties were involved, because the plans did not have the same benefits, rates, or contract forms—three elements necessary for reciprocity. The differences reflected local conditions, and there were differing ideas of what benefits ought to be provided under the reciprocity agreement, and how it should be managed. Only about half the plans ever accepted the agreement, and it began to break down almost as soon as it had been adopted. One at a time, the basic elements were removed from the reciprocity agreement and replaced by detailed contractual commitments among the plans which spelled out exactly what was to be done and how.

First to be revised was the system for providing benefits for a member in the hospital away from home. This may have been tackled first because more money was involved than in the other reciprocal efforts. Besides, somebody had an idea of how to correct the inequities. Originally, if a Maine plan subscriber was hospitalized in Massachusetts, for example, Massachusetts would try to allow hospital services as close as possible to what the subscriber was entitled to get in Maine. But the Massachusetts plan would have to pay the Massachusetts hospital at Massachusetts cost levels, then Maine would reimburse the Massachusetts plan. It didn't work. Massachusetts did not fully understand Maine benefits; sometimes the Maine member was no longer a paid-up member when he was in the hospital, and there was no procedure to find out about his status while he was still hospitalized. Further, hospital care cost more in Massachusetts, and Maine could not afford it, although Massachusetts was happy when the situation was reversed.

Paul A. Webb, executive director of the plan in Portland, Maine, proposed a reformulation of this approach in 1946. Rorem assigned the project to Antone G. Singsen, then assistant director of the commission office, who organized a series of economic and administrative studies, formed a committee of plan-operating people, and developed a new program known as the Inter-Plan Service Benefit Bank. The "bank" began operations in 1949 and, with modifications over the years, has continued in effect up to the present time. Webb's concept was to set up a sort of clearing house (he first called it a bank) to administer days of care which each plan would buy at its own average local cost, and would use everywhere else in the country whenever one of its members was hospitalized. The benefits to be provided would be those of the "host" plan, whose member hospitals knew what they were and therefore could make proper credit. The host plan would be paid its own cost by the clearing house. All this was expected to balance out financially between high cost and low cost plans. The concept was sound administratively, but high and low cost plans did not balance out. Since more members then belonged to high cost plans, and a lot of away-from-home care was provided in low cost plans, the bank would have collected too much money. Singsen and his committee tested formulas, wrote rules, and ultimately hit on a balance under which low cost plans like Maine paid a little more than their local cost of care and plans like Massachusetts paid less than their local cost, and everybody was happy—including the members, who got their benefits, and the hospitals, which did not have to deal with plans outside their contractual agreements. All the plans joined the bank in a few years.

Having solved one part of the original reciprocity problem, the commission assigned Singsen to tackle a second part—transfer of members who moved residence or employment from one plan area to another. The trick was to develop a transfer method without the transferred member's having to go through a period of temporary coverage exclusions or waiting periods, or meet local underwriting regulations. The same process of identifying problems and developing compromise administrative solutions proved successful again, and a New Inter-Plan Transfer Agreement went into effect in 1951. The key problem was that population was flowing in every-increasing numbers to the so-called sunshine states such as Florida, California, and Arizona; and since many of the Blue Cross members who wanted to transfer were at somewhat advanced ages and sometimes were moving because of ill health as well, those particular Blue Cross plans were being asked to take on high risk, potentially high cost subscribers—thus distorting the average mix resulting from purely local sales efforts. Also, only those members who asked for a change were transferred, so that the original plan tended to keep the good risks and lose the bad risks, while the new plan got only the latter. Also, not all plans had by then adopted sound underwriting regulations, and those plans which felt they did have good rules were not happy to have to accept members from plans which did not. Again, the committee promulgated regulations to deal with all these problems, produce a greater degree of equity, and allow the sunshine state plans to handle their special problems a little differently from the way the other plans handled theirs. Once again, all plans agreed to the Inter-Plan Transfer Agreement in a short time, and that program also has continued to work, with modifications, up to the present.

The problem of enrolling employees in nationwide industries cutting across several states was more difficult. Much more cooperation was needed among plans for this type of enrollment when uniformity of benefits and procedures was demanded by the prospective account. Primarily, each plan geared its enrollment policies and procedures to its own area only, and it was a complicated and sensitive matter to come up with a single way to deal with a big account when each plan wanted to have one administrative procedure and one set of benefits apply to everything. The problem of national enrollment will be discussed in detail in another chapter; it was a central issue in the Blue Cross movement over many years. But the effort to do something about it was the third part of the original 1944 reciprocity program.

After developing the bank and transfer programs, the enrollment procedure was also refashioned to develop a common approach toward some national accounts when uniformity of benefits was not required. A so-called Consolidated Billing Agreement set up some administrative rules for handling multiplan accounts. In 1953 this was replaced by a Local Benefits Agreement for National Accounts, with more specific rules requiring some concessions by local plans as to acceptable forms, performance on delivery of identification cards, notices of rate changes, and related matters. This program did not solve the problems of who was to be responsible for the account, what levels of benefit were to be proposed, or what to do if uniform benefits or rates were needed. But if the account would accept a series of local variations fitting each of the communities in which it was located, the Local Benefits Agreement provided some rules for handling it. Many large accounts, such as the automobile companies, operated in this manner for many years. The first attempt to set up a national sales office also came in this period. Van Dyk was engaged by the commission as part-time manager of a national enrollment office located in New York, where he was then chief marketing executive of the New York City plan.

As early as 1942 the Blue Cross leadership was convinced that hospital care benefits alone were only a partial solution to the risks of costly medical episodes facing families. A parallel medical service prepayment plan was necessary to round out the benefit package and encourage sales. The medical society–sponsored physician service plans had barely started at this time, and their rapid expansion was to come later. In the 1940s, efforts were being made by several Blue Cross plans to get companion surgical-medical benefits to supplement hospital care benefits. In some places, Blue Cross plans added their own surgical-medical benefits, primarily physicians' services in the hospital, on an indemnity basis, with no contract with physicians. Other Blue Cross plans helped to start companion corporations. The problem of national accounts led to several of these efforts to get medical benefits.

Stuart reports that in 1942 he, J. Douglas Colman of Baltimore, and Frank Deniston of Chicago met in Baltimore with representatives of the Commercial Credit Company, and they were successful in obtaining a capital fund of $150,000. Benefits and enrollment rates were formulated, and the American Health Insurance Company was launched. The sole purpose was to write companion surgical-medical benefits for Blue Cross plans.[4] Deniston was made vice-president on a two year contract. He set up an office and waited for business from the Blue Cross plans, which Stuart reported were enthusiastically in favor of the project. But, "No business came—none at all." After the next annual meeting of the Blue Cross plans, Commercial Credit Company adjusted Deniston's contract and paid him off.[5] Blue Cross plans were clearly not ready for this kind of venture. There was suspicion of private, for-profit insurance company ventures, and fear that Blue Cross plans might lose control in this formative period of their development.

Another early effort to solve the problem of physicians' service benefits concerned Louis H. Pink in 1943, when he became chairman of the board of the New York City plan still headed by Frank Van Dyk. Pink tried to induce 10 Blue Cross plans to put up $50,000 each to establish an insurance company which would sell insurance covering surgical-medical services. It appears that the Blue Cross plan executives involved agreed, but they were unable to persuade their respective boards to put up the money. The proposal failed.[6] Again, Blue Cross plans were not ready. However, this important matter of surgical-medical benefits and national accounts could not rest.

Mannix was very impatient with the Blue Cross plans' failure to move. As early as 1940 he had proposed a national organization to offer Blue Cross benefits on a nationwide basis to national employees. He said, "They nearly threw me out of the Blue Cross movement the first time I presented it in October, 1940 . . ."[7] He was then executive director of the Michigan plan. From 1940 to 1946 he kept pushing for a national program, both openly and behind the scenes, but he was far ahead of the inclinations of other Blue Cross plan directors. The next splash came in the form of a proposal in 1944, when he was director of the Chicago plan, for the hospitals and the medical profession to get together to establish an "American Blue Cross" plan offering a combined package of hospital and physicians' services to national accounts through local Blue Cross plans. Mannix proposed that this agency should acquire a national charter from Congress analogous to that of the American Red Cross. A prestigious board of directors should be appointed made up of hospital, medical, and public representatives. He felt that only by so doing could the voluntary

---

[4]James E. Stuart, "The Blue Cross History: An Informal Biography of the Voluntary Non-Profit Prepayment Plan for Hospital Care" (Unpublished manuscript, 1960). p. 10.

[5]The American Health Insurance Company, however, continued under new management and reorganized to sell health insurance as a private insurance company, in effect becoming a competitor of Blue Cross plans.

[6]Taped telephone conversation between Singsen and Mannix, February 26, 1974.

[7]Interview in Cleveland, February 24, 1971.

method and philosophy of meeting the family costs of health services succeed. The national plan would embody all the original Blue Cross principles, i.e., nonprofit, service benefits, community rate, and noncompeting jurisdictions. A startling suggestion for the time was that the rate should be based on subscriber incomes, and that there should be some subsidy for the unemployed. Even though Mannix regarded Blue Cross as an agent of the public, he still had faith in a large measure of provider control of voluntary health insurance enterprise and its ability and desire to operate in the public interest. In any case, Mannix' plan received only passing attention, in articles published in the official journal of the American Hospital Association, *Hospitals,*[8] and the *Journal of the American Medical Association*. Blue Cross plans, even if they had been willing to act concertedly, an unlikely possibility at that time, could not possibly bring in physicians' services. Medical society–sponsored physician prepayment plans were neither strong nor ready.

Two years later, Mannix made a much more dramatic and personally serious and courageous move by resigning from the Chicago plan to head up a stock company, the John Marshall Insurance Co., to sell national accounts. He was approached by a group of people in Huntington, West Virginia, to undertake this task through the newly formed company, and completely separate himself from the Blue Cross movement. He immediately became a renegade in the eyes of his Blue Cross confreres—especially, perhaps, because he was chairman of the commission at that time. In the Blue Cross view he had acquired the taint of the profit approach to hospital care insurance, and he had no hospital backing. Mannix wanted it in the record that he had stipulated he would accept the job only if the profits of the company were limited to *one* percent of gross income. Surprisingly, the investors had agreed to this, but the venture proved to be a disaster and lasted only two years.[9] The corporation was sold to the Bankers' Life and Casualty Co. in Chicago. As it turned out, an old friend and associate from his Cleveland days, John McNamara, resigned from the Cleveland Blue Cross plan at about that time, and Mannix was offered the executive directorship of that plan in 1948; he remained there until his retirement in 1965. Gradually, he regained the regard of his Blue Cross peers and again become active in the voluntary nonprofit health insurance movement.

Mannix' characteristically lone and swashbuckling style was not

[8] John R. Mannix, "Why Not an American Blue Cross?" *Hospitals*, April, 1944. (Reprint)

[9] Mannix believed the company would have been successful if it had not encountered a rapid rise in hospital costs. In 24 months the hospital per diem increased from $7 to $12: "We could not raise our rates fast enough to take care of this marked inflation." It should be observed that Blue Cross plans faced the same increase in hospital per diem rates as Mannix' company, and they survived.

compatible with the need for a gradual convergence of national and local actions; the balancing of both forces was necessary to make Blue Cross fully effective. The national Blue Cross leadership continued to be restive. Some means had to be found to handle national accounts. It is a tribute to the leadership that Blue Cross continued to grow in spite of this persistent unsolved problem.

Chapter Seven

Beginning to Get Together

At the end of 1946, Rorem resigned as executive director of the Blue Cross Plan Commission, a post he had held for 10 years. There were several reasons. Certainly he must have been discouraged with the abortive attempts to unify the plans. The service benefit was being eroded. There was some internal strife. He was then over 50 years of age, and probably restless. Moreover, a new opportunity beckoned which would engage his wider interests—the planning of the supply side of hospital care, rather than the financing of supply on a periodic basis. He went to Philadelphia to head the Hospital Planning Council there.

The public relations director he had hired, Richard M. Jones, became acting executive director and permanent director within a year. Antone Singsen, whom Rorem also had hired, became assistant director. The name of the national body was changed to the Blue Cross Commission. Both Jones and Singsen were originally trained as journalists. Jones was new to Blue Cross plans; Singsen had been with Blue Cross sincd 1939, starting in the Rhode Island plan.

In Rorem's last report to the Blue Cross Plan Commission in December 1946, he wrote: "Blue Cross and medical plans are important examples of enlightened self-interest on the part of the public, the medical profession, and the hospitals in which important health services are performed. There are also examples of self-discipline, which is the price of self-determination. The task is hard, but the rewards justify the effort." There is no hint here that Rorem felt the Blue Cross idea was in the clear and running, nor that the then emerging medical society Blue Shield plans were going to sweep the field. Thirteen years later when Rorem was given the Justin Ford Kimball Award by the American Hospital Association for meritorious service to hospital prepayment, he said: "Many people were convinced that group payment for hospital service was unsound. One important national group first thought it was unethical, later that it was illegal, finally, that it was impossible."[1]

The group referred to was obviously the American Medical Association, but the American Hospital Association was not exactly a leader in hospital prepayment, either, until local plans had shown the way and some outside money from the Rosenwald Fund had helped to start the national agency. AHA acted only after local groups had started a common characteristic of federations. Nor did AHA provide any money for continuation of the commission after the Rosenwald grant was terminated.

In 1937, state medical societies had sponsored physicians' service plans in California, Michigan, and Pennsylvania. Precursors of these were the county medical bureaus in the state of Washington, organized in the 1930s to counteract contract medicine, and later to ward off the threat of universal health insurance. Still later, these bureaus served another function by competing with the group practice prepayment started by Kaiser Industries on the West Coast.

By 1946 there were 43 medical society plans and a nationwide enrollment of three million. In that year the American Medical Association contributed $25,000 to establish the Associated Medical Care Plans, the analogue to the Blue Cross Commission. From the start, there emerged on the surface a cooperative relationship between the Blue Cross Commission and the Associated Medical Care Plans, which eventually became the National Association of Blue Shield Plans. Below the surface, only periodically breaking into the open, the relationship had its tensions and conflicts. The issue was how to unify Blue Cross hospital benefits and Blue Shield physician benefits without either group becoming dominant over the other, the chronic hospital-physician struggle. The AMA hierarchy never backed the Blue Shield plans unreservedly, and the desired unified Blue Cross and Blue Shield benefit package remained out of reach. Still, the two groups related to each other somehow, achieving some cooperation, at least, in sales.

After Rorem's departure, the Blue Cross plans did not appear to want to strengthen the central organization, and the commission was weak as a unifying national force. Jones was temperamentally suited to a moderator's role, as Rorem certainly was not, and he also realized that for the time being, at least, the plans did not want a strong national organization. Jones sensed perceptively that the real leadership had to come from the plan directors themselves rather than from the commission. He tried to have Blue Cross function through a large number of committees representing various activities and concepts of what

---

[1] C. Rufus Rorem, "Hospital Care a Community Affair: The Justin Ford Kimball Award Address." Blue Cross Program Session, April 13, 1959, p. 18.

should be done: "He did not aspire to leadership, but rather to attempt to keep peace in the Blue Cross family."[2] Jones was director for 13 years, until 1960, and within his perceived role served the Blue Cross idea well, but also, as he himself realized, more national unity was needed. He lived with a great deal of ferment.

For a diffusion of power, and to decrease the influence of AHA, the Blue Cross plans in 1947 set up 11 geographic districts (12 including Canada), with one plan director elected as commissioner for each district. Each plan in a district, regardless of size, had one vote for commissioner. The district system lasted until 1957. According to Stuart, the chairmanship of the commission was passed from one plan director to another as an honor, and as something to be expected in due course "It was a democratic method but not one that always assured inspired or even enlightened leadership in the building of national programs."[3]

Still, some remarkably aggressive and foresighted men were champing at the bit to achieve national unity. The Inter-Plan Service Benefit Bank was an example. The chief problem, however, continued to be some form of national enrollment for national accounts that would be competitive with private insurance companies and help expand Blue Cross as a national entity. The national enrollment office limped along, inadequately funded and inadequately staffed, but the idea of a national enrollment mechanism would not die.

In another effort to create a strong national enrollment program several plans in 1947 formulated what became known as the syndicate. This imaginative idea is attributed to van Steenwyk, who had moved from Minnesota to head the Philadelphia plan. The basic concept was to have a Blue Cross plan which was in the same area as the home office of a company with branches in more than one state write a uniform contract for this company for all areas where it had employees. The Blue Cross plan which had jurisdiction in the home office area would then grant power of attorney to the other Blue Cross plans involved. Since the benefits and rates negotiated by the first Blue Cross plan would not be similar to the benefits and rates of the cooperating plans, these plans would then have to write contracts tailored to the original specifications, so as to have uniform benefits everywhere. The Philadelphia plan first enrolled the American Viscose Corporation under the syndicate arrangement. Shortly thereafter, the Pittsburgh plan headed by Abraham Oseroff and the Chicago plan under Robert T. Evans used the same device; United States Steel, Bethlehem

---

[2]James E. Stuart, "The Blue Cross History: An Informal Biography of the Voluntary Non-Profit Prepayment Plan for Hospital Care" (Unpublished manuscript, 1966), p. 149.

[3]Ibid, p. 150.

Steel, and the Jewel Tea Company were the big enrollment prizes. In five years the syndicate method produced 250 syndicates and an enrollment of over one million members.[4] The successor to Oseroff at the Pittsburgh plan, William H. Ford, regarded the syndicate idea as one of the most significant enrollment breakthroughs in Blue Cross history.[5] At last, it permitted a combination of Blue Cross plans to work together effectively on one enrollment contract, although as a side effect it may have contributed something to erosion of the community rate concept, to be replaced by merit or experience rating. Once an enrollment contract cut across plans with different benefits, rates, and hospital utilization patterns, the community rate became untenable. Each plan in the syndicate kept track of its own experience and reported it to the head plan.

Blue Cross leadership, however, did not feel that the syndicate method of enrolling national accounts by itself would meet the problem.[6] Blue Cross leaders periodically were shocked by the loss of large national contracts to private insurance companies. At a meeting of the Blue Cross Commission in Milwaukee in April 1947, Louis H. Pink, by this time president of the New York City plan, proposed that the Blue Cross Commission set up a membership corporation to handle national enrollment. The commission voted to explore this possibility. Significantly, Frank E. Smith, director of the Associated Medical Care Plans, the federation of medical society–sponsored prepayment plans, was present at the meeting and suggested that the commission consider writing to his agency recommending that it participate in the exploration.[7] On the staff level, Jones for the Blue Cross Commission and Smith for AMCP had established cooperative relations. The Council on Medical Service of the AMA was reported to be willing to cooperate in sharing information and data "but still retains too favorable an attitude toward commercial health insurance."[8]

The Blue Cross Commission moved rapidly. William S. McNary, who that year had moved to the Michigan plan from Colorado, was appointed to chair a special committee on a national enrollment corporation. By the next meeting of the blue Cross Commission, held in St. Louis in September 1947, he presented the following recommendatons, which were unanimously adopted:

> That the Blue Cross Commission proceed to establish a membership corporation, the members of which shall be voluntary, non-profit hospital and *medical plans* (emphasis added), to perform the services necessary in the enrollment of national accounts and to engage in

[4]Ibid, p. 192.
[5]Interview in Chicago, March 24, 1973.
[6]Stuart, "The Blue Cross History," p. 194.
[7]Blue Cross Commission, Minutes, Milwaukee, April 19–21, 1947.
[8]Ibid.

such other activities as shall strengthen the entire voluntary, non-profit health care movement.[9]

Selected functions of the membership corporation were described:

1. Contract with subscribing groups on behalf of plans.
2. Contract with plans and receive proper authorization from them to enter into contracts and carry on business with subscribing groups.
3. Establish central billing and collect and distribute funds to plans.
4. Contract with plans for provisions of service benefits in all areas through an Inter-Plan Service Benefit Bank or its equivalent.
5. Provide protection for members of subscribing groups in areas where arrangements cannot be made with local plans, through the establishment of a nonprofit insurance corporation which shall be wholly owned by the membership corporation (i.e., the Blue Cross Commission). (The significance of this was obvious: to bypass laggard local plans if necessary.)

Other recommendations were that the nonprofit insurance corporation should be adequately funded to assure long-term stability; the board of trustees should be small, and the majority of its members should be board members of the participating plans. The Blue Cross Commission was instructed to draft a proposed membership corporation charter and bylaws and a plan of incorpation for acceptance by the plans. Further, and significantly, the administrator selected to head the membership corporation as its chief administrative officer should be from outside present Blue Cross and medical plan paid administrative personnel. There was to be a search for a new leader free of previous entanglements and imputed vested interests in hospital and medical prepayment development. Finally, the Blue Cross Commission was to invite the Associated Medical Care Plans Commission to cooperate in the implementation of these recommendations. Such a unified approach, it was believed, would strengthen the voluntary health insurance movement immeasurably.

After the Blue Cross Commission had adopted these recommendations, and during the course of the same commission meeting, there was a joint meeting of the Blue Cross and the AMCP commissions to discuss the possibility of cooperation. It was a portentous meeting; the brass on both the hospital and medical sides were out in full force. The atmosphere was strained but negotiable. Dr. F. L. Feierabend of the AMCP board was asked to preside. Feierabend had

[9]Blue Cross Commission, Minutes, St. Louis, September 19–20, 1947.

been a long-time, dedicated promoter of medical prepayment within the AMA and was a charter member of the AMCP board. In opening the meeting he declared that it was a truly historic occasion, "boding well for the future of voluntary prepayment plans."[10]

Feierabend called on Frank Van Dyk of New York to comment on the problems of national enrollment and the desirability of combining hospital and medical-surgical benefits. Van Dyk stated realistically that the inclusion of medical benefits was especially difficult because of the lack of nationwide coverage by medical plans and the variation in medical plan contracts. He urged that efforts be made to standardize both Blue Cross and medical-surgical benefits and procedures.

The immediate and modest result of this joint meeting was recognition by the commission members of the necessity for their staffs to establish capabilities for obtaining information and data needed by both commissions, and to make use of the research facilities of the AMA.[11] Between September and December 1947, the two commissions came to an agreement on a candidate for the position of chief executive officer of the proposed membership corporation that was to coordinate the activities of the Blue Cross Commission and the AMCP Commission. There was also agreement on how the salary would be shared, considering that Blue Cross plans at that time had a much larger income than the medical plans. The chief executive officer would be expected to work out details of the proposed national membership and national enrollment organizations.[12]

The person selected to become the chief executive officer was Paul R. Hawley, M.D., Major General, U.S. Army Medical Corps, Retired former chief surgeon, European Theater of Operations, World War II, and at that time the medical director of the U.S. Veterans Administration. He was clearly regarded as a leader, and equally clearly, hospital and medical prepayment needed a leader to pull the factions together in the interests of the providers and the public. At a joint meeting of the Blue Cross and Blue Shield Commissions (now changed from AMCP), in Washington, D.C., on December 22, 1947, formal action was

---

[10]In an interview with Feierabend on August 31, 1971, in Kansas City he revealed himself to be the complete physician and human being. He was one of a handful of prominent physicians throughout the country who backed the medical prepayment movement. He said he was motivated by the Catholic doctrine of subsidiarity: Wherever there is a social problem, it becomes a responsibility of the lower (i.e., lower than the state) and better qualified group—in this case, organized medicine. He said: "The AMA hierarchy was unalterably opposed to Blue Cross and Blue Shield." He was never put on a single committee when he was in the AMA House of Delegates. Feierabend died in 1972.

[11]Joint Meeting of the Blue Cross Commission and the AMCP Commission, Minutes, St. Louis, September 20, 1947.

[12]Blue Cross Commission, Minutes, Chicago, December 13, 1947.

taken to hire Hawley effective January 1, 1948.[13] He was given the title of chief executive officer; Richard M. Jones, director of the Blue Cross Commission, and Frank E. Smith, director of the AMCP Commission, reported to Hawley, and he reported to a joint executive committee. The two commissions had thereby committed themselves in principle, although neither yet had the official backing of its provider association. The American Hospital Association and the American Medical Association, presumably, were expected to approve the actions that had already been taken. Hawley's contract was for one year.

During the first half of 1948, the Blue Cross Commission sought to acquaint member plans with the implications of a national membership corporation. There was the inevitable trepidation about delegation of powers to a central agency. At a meeting of the Blue Cross Commission in Los Angeles in March, the plans were assured that a national corporation (1) would not cost plans more (no increase in dues), (2) would not disturb the plan district system, (3) would not jeopardize local plan autonomy, and (4) would not change the weighted vote basis of determining action on all matters (a sensitive issue among "small" plans).[14]

The crucial meeting occurred in Chicago on June 17, 1948. Another veteran leader, Dr. Basil C. MacLean, who threads through the early history of hospital prepayment, had been chairman of a special committee to review the proposal for a national service agency for action at this meeting; this agency was to be known as Blue Cross and Blue Shield Health Service, Inc. Its board of directors would consist of 15 members from Blue Cross and 15 from Blue Shield. The recommendation was adopted,[15] and, again, the board of trustees of the American Hospital Association subsequently approved the action. It was now AMA's turn to show its hand, and so it did—to the consternation of many.

Blue Cross and Blue Shield representatives at the staff level had been having a series of meetings, with McNary of Michigan as the spokesman for Blue Cross, and Jay Ketchum of Michigan Blue Shield acting for Blue Shield. McNary and Ketchum had an excellent working relationship in the Michigan plans, and it was possible, at least, that this would influence the national groups.[16] According to Stuart, Blue Cross representatives arrived at a complete agreement, and a minority of the Blue Shield representatives, led by Ketchum, arrived at the same agreement for establishment of an organization to be called Health Services, Inc.,

[13]Joint Blue Cross Commission and Blue Shield Commission meeting, Minutes, Washington, D.C., December 22, 1947.
[14]Blue Cross Commission, Minutes, Los Angeles, March 26, 1948.
[15]Blue Cross Commission, Minutes, Chicago, June 17, 1948.
[16]Interview with Jay Ketchum in Ft. Lauderdale, Florida, March 23, 1973. He said, for example, that he and McNary never asked each other for anything unless it was absolutely necessary for the advancement or survival of their respective plans.

proposed to give the national management, under Hawley, the instrument needed to carry out the national task.

It was apparent that the Blue Cross Commission by its action of June 17 was testing the ultimate intentions of AMA. Later, the Council on Medical Service of AMA opposed the proposal for Blue Cross and Blue Shield Health Service, Inc. The house of delegates of AMA at its interim session on November 30, 1948, upheld this recommendation, and the joint venture foundered. Then Blue Shield plans also voted "no," and it was dead.

What were the reasons? As usual, there were several. The legal reason given was AMA's fear of restraint of trade action which might result from hospital and physician cooperation of this nature. Another reason was the fear that a joint national insurance agency would be controlled by Blue Cross, which was the larger and, for all its divisiveness, the more cohesive organization. As it was expressed by Feierabend of Blue Shield, a physician sympathetic to the joint effort: "The Blue Cross group was saying, 'I'm not going to let any doctor tell us how to run a hospital.' The Blue Shield group was saying, 'I'm not going to let any guy who doesn't know anything about medicine tell me how to practice.' So there you were; there was the clash."[17]

Naturally, the action of AMA was a blow to the prestige of Hawley, who was counted on to bridge the gap between hospitals and physicians. The plausible interpretation is that the underlying differences between hospital prepayment and medical prepayment were so profound and controversial that no "great man" could transcend the gulf. Blue Cross and hospital administrators automatically think in terms of systems; physicians, with only rare exceptions, feel threatened by administrative structures and systems. The Blue Cross idea was a vanguard and expanding enterprise. Blue Cross directors had a favorable fusion of motives—personal ambition in an expanding enterprise hitched to a statistically demonstrable need for some type of prepayment for the large, self-sustaining element of the population. Blue Shield, in the view of its critics, admitted the need for prepayment grudgingly; it was made available rather than promoted aggressively. Symbolically, the national office of AMA had enrolled its own employees in private insurance companies rather than Blue Shield and Blue Cross.

Nevertheless, Blue Shield plans now began to expand rapidly. John Castellucci of Michigan, who succeeded Frank E. Smith as the director of the national Blue Shield office, made the following observation. He was asked: "When the chips were down, how reliable do you feel the medical profession was in backing you up?" Castellucci answered: "If you're speaking of the profession, the individual physician as opposed to the hierarchy in medicine, I say when the

17Interview, Kansas City, Missouri, August 31, 1971.

chips were down we got wonderful support. Unfortunately, it didn't at all times carry through the hierarchy in the politics of medicine, because in the nature of the beast, the politician plays all sides,"[18] Castellucci observed further that 80 percent of practicing physicians were signed up with plans in their areas. In any case, the national Blue Cross and Blue Shield agencies went ahead without AMA support and set up their own corporations for national enrollment purposes.

The Blue Cross Commission established its own agency, Health Services, Inc. This was a stock insurance company, chartered in Illinois, to be operated on a nonprofit basis and authorized to write health, accident, and all forms of casualty insurance. The stock was to be owned by the Blue Cross plans. To provide for stock ownership it was necessary legally to organize a nonprofit corporation also chartered in Illinois, known as the Blue Cross Association.[19] Hawley became president of the corporation; Oseroff was treasurer, Jones secretary, and Singsen assistant secretary and assistant treasurer. It was a paper corporation. On the original board there were four plan directors, seven plan board members, and two Blue Cross Commission employees. Two people not connected with Blue Cross were appointed, Mrs. Agnes E. Meyer of the *Washington Post* and the late Walter P. Reuther, president of United Automobile Workers. Robert N. Rose, a New York insurance executive, was appointed president of Health Service, Inc. in January 1950. HSI was to operate as a national enrollment office and as an underwriter to fill benefit gaps in national contracts and thus level out the peaks and valleys in benefits among plans.

Simultaneously, Blue Shield organized a medical counterpart to Health Service, Inc., eventually known as Medical Indemnity of America (MIA). Three years later, in 1953, HSO and MIA formulated a joint operating agreement. All underwriting was to be undertaken jointly, each company insuring 50 percent of the risk and assuming one-half of the administrative cost.[20] Neither HSI by itself nor HSI and MIA jointly were outstandingly successful in enrolling national accounts. By 1954, only 31 of the 83 Blue Cross plans in the United States had agreed to write the standard HIA-MIA hospital contract. After four years of joint HSI-MIA activity, the two agencies had 361 groups and 500,000 or so subscribers.[21] This could scarcely be regarded as strong competition for the private insurance companies, which by that time were counting policyholders in millions.

[18] Interview in Ft. Lauderdale, March 23, 1973.
[19] There were other reasons for creation of the Blue Cross Association besides the need to own the stock of HSI. The Blue Cross Commission was frequently faced with the need to do something outside the scope of AHA bylaws. Examples are the National Retirement Program, a trusted retirement plan for employees of participating plans with BCA; and the switching of a master agreement with the Bell System from BCC to BCA so that its retirees could be enrolled.
[20] Stuart, "The Blue Cross History," p. 203.
[21] Ibid, p. 205.

Around 1950, an insurance company actuary, Edmund C. Whittaker of Prudential, invented the major medical concept. J. Albert Durgom of New Jersey Blue Cross regarded this concept as brilliant from the private insurance companies' standpoint, offering as it did an attractively low premium for protection beyond Blue Cross–Blue Shield benefits as the deductible.[22] HSI and MIA were the natural instruments for Blue Cross and Blue Shield plans to write national major medical accounts on top of their own basic benefits, but according to Stuart the plans concentrated their efforts instead on major medical contracts in their local plans rather than nationally.

Despite these seemingly modest attainments during the period from 1948 to 1952, which Stuart liked to call a "golden age" in Blue Cross development, Blue Cross plans did establish a framework for national coordination. This was a time when Colman was chairman of the commission for two years and McNary the next two years; Hawley was appointed during Colman's chairmanship. These were the years when the Inter-Plan Service Benefit Bank and Health Services, Inc. were established, both of great importance for the national stance of Blue Cross plans. Hawley remained for less than three years and then left to become director of the American College of Surgeons. Even though he did not attain the hoped for Blue Cross and Blue Shield unification, his presence was helpful in the effort to mold Blue Cross plans into a national entity. Although the instruments were there, dissatisfaction with their operation continued. Consequently, during the latter part of the 1950s, the Blue Cross Commission and Blue Cross Association reorganized and emerged as the BCA that exists today.

While Blue Cross plans were occupied with all these internal conflicts and growth problems, the possibility of some form of universal health insurance in the United States remained in the background. From the groups at interest—American Hospital Association, American Medical Association, hospitals, physicians, Blue Cross and Blue Shield plans, and private insurance companies—there came the repeated refrain: "If we do not do the job government will do it for us." The threat gave the various factions in voluntary health insurance a negative incentive for achieving unity, albeit a very ragged unity up to this time.

Unless one was an adult during the 1940s, it is difficult to believe that the polemical battles between the proponents of voluntary health insurance and government health insurance were as intense as actually was the case. Self-righteousness characterized all the groups, not least the AMA hierarchy and the proponents of government health insurance. The temper of the times was

[22] Interview, Chicago, January 3, 1973.

exemplified during a conference on health insurance sponsored by the Bureau of Public Health Economics, School of Public Health, University of Michigan, in Ann Arbor, in 1944. This conference brought all the interested groups together in one place, perhaps for the first time. The big names of representative Blue Cross and Blue Shield plans, private insurance companies, and government were there. I was then on the staff of the university's Bureau of Public Health Economics and heard the debates between the voluntary and government proponents, which were intense and at times bordered on hostility. Van Steenwyk wanted private insurance companies and government to stay out of health insurance altogether and leave the field to Blue Cross and Blue Shield plans, where the responsibility properly belonged, in his mind. I. S. Falk, then of the Social Security Administration, predicted that voluntary health insurance would shortly reach its enrollment limit and be found inadequate. Although he had favored the voluntary approach in the early thirties, he soon began to feel that the "force of law needed to be used on the financing side, although not on the supply side."[23] The battle lines were clarifying on several issues, both internal and external to the voluntary health insurance agencies.

During the forties, Blue Cross plans tried hard to differentiate themselves from private insurance companies, not to mention staying clear of government health insurance, by establishing a terminology distinctive to Blue Cross. Blue Shield plans were much less unified on this point, because the medical profession was ambiguous toward its own plans. The American Medical Association chose to recognize the nonprofit and private insurance company approaches simultaneously.

Blue Cross executives preferred to use terms such as "members" rather than "policyholders," "rates" rather than "premiums," "service" rather than "indemnity," "enrolling" rather than "selling," and "enrollment representatives" rather than "salesmen." The most militant advocate of such a pure terminology was Stuart of the Cincinnati plan. He had arrived on the scene relatively late, in 1942, but he quickly moved into prominence and became the "conscience" of Blue Cross, fulfilling a role Rorem had played earlier. A lawyer by training, Stuart came to Blue Cross from a significant career in public welfare administration and community work.

One of Rorem's last public acts as director of the Blue Cross Commission was to testify before the U.S. Senate Committee on Education and Labor in April 1946, on Senate Bill 1606, relating to a comprehensive government health insurance proposal. As was the policy of the Blue Cross Commission and the American Hospital Association at that time, Rorem

[23]Interview, New Haven, Conn., April 2, 1971.

recommended grants-in-aid to states to be applied to low income families for enrollment in Blue Cross plans. One of the senators asked: ". . . and you are not advocating . . . the creating of a compulsory health insurance plan?" Rorem replied, "You are entirely correct. In fact, I would go further and say not only are we not advocating it, but we would regard that as a last step to take, from our point of view, at the present stage of the organization of health service, a premature step."[24]   The federal government should help make the voluntary approach work, not replace it.

Proponents of government health insurance were dubious. Still, the U.S. Public Health Service, through a health economist on its staff, Louis S. Reed, who initiated the idea, suggested to Blue Cross and Blue Shield plans that a study be made of their status and operations. Reed had been a staff member of the Committee on the Costs of Medical Care, where he knew Rorem. He had been on Falk's staff in the Social Security Administration, but in 1939 he had moved to the public health methods section of the Public Health Servcie under George St. J. Perrott, a well-known health service statistician. Although Reed had published a book in 1937 in which he recommended government health insurance,[25]   he was open-minded enough to look into the growing voluntary health insurance plans. Reed had started to visit Blue Cross plans as early as 1938, starting with Cleveland which was then administered by John McNamara. "It was very interesting, and I was impressed with what I saw."[26]   In time, Reed felt that the Blue Cross and Blue Shield plans warranted thorough study. He broached this possibility in 1944 to Rorem, who was reported to be quite enthusiastic. Later, Reed sold the idea to Perrott, and in due course, a formal request came to the commission from Surgeon General Thomas Parran. Reed said that "it took a fair amount of doing" to persuade the Blue Cross people, who were suspicious. It is likely that they were flattered by the attention and recognition and at the same time wary of the motives of an agency whose health experts were known to favor government insurance. The idea had to be sold both on the commission level and to all the individual plans. Van Steenwyk was sympathetic and cautious. Eventually the proposal was approved at a meeting with the big plan leaders in New York. "I was nervous as a cub," Reed reported. He and his associate, Henry Vaughan, Jr., later visited many of the plans and collected extensive data on all of them, and a detailed, informative, and straightforward book was published by the U.S. Public Health Service in 1947.[27]

24 As reproduced in Blue Cross Commission, "Self-Portrait," 1946, p. 25.
25 Louis S. Reed, *Health Insurance: The Next Step in Social Security* (New York: Harper, 1937).
26 Interview in McLean, Virginia, February 7, 1971.
27 Louis S. Reed, *Blue Cross and Medical Service Plans* (Washington: Federal Security Agency, Public Health Service, 1947), p. 323.

Reed was favorably impressed with the plan directors, their enthusiasm, and the apparent potential of the Blue Cross development: ". . . there was an enthusiasm about the people in the early plans; it was very catching. They felt that they were great pioneers, and they were. . . . It was all an enjoyable experience, and it thrilled me, and the guys were pleasant to be with, and they were good people. They were devoted." Reed's assessment did not sit well with his colleagues in the government. He was getting a longer range perspective than his colleagues had: ". . . the news that I was bringing back was generally news that they didn't want to hear. I was saying, 'Fellows, look, this is big. These plans are developing, and they are going to be a big thing. You have to take that into account.' It was unwelcome news."[28] In fact, Reed had problems getting the report finished and approved. He was accused of selling out. Perrott, however, did not feel that Reed had gone off the deep end, as others did.

These and other behind-the-scenes struggles illustrated the early emergence of countervailing forces in the health service, prepayment, and insurance fields. Civil servants were hardly a neutral group. A series of proposals for government-sponsored national health insurance got as far as bill form in Congress, but none of them reached the floor for a showdown debate. When Truman was president he tried hard to get such legislation enacted; failing, he regarded it later as one of his unfinished tasks.[29] Truman's secretary of the Federal Security Agency (later the Department of Health, Education, and Welfare), Oscar Ewing, predicted in 1948 that voluntary health insurance would probably never be able to cover more than one-half the population.[30] He was not alone in this prediction, but the source is significant.

Truman made a statesmanlike move in 1951 in establishing the President's Commission on the Health Needs of the Nation, by means of a congressional appropriation entitled Emergency Fund for the President, National Defense. Under the umbrella of national preparedness the president could authorize such a commission. Truman took great pains to make certain that commission members had complete freedom to make public policy recommendations regarding health service, regardless of whether or not they agreed with the known policies of his administration. He appointed an impressive group representing the public, organized labor, medicine, dentistry, nursing, and hospitals. Chairman of the commission was Paul B. Magnuson, M.D., a distinguished orthopedic surgeon who was professor emeritus at Northwestern University Medical School, Chicago. The report proved to be a benchmark of the status of the health services field, summarizing and organizing the relevant

[28] Interview, February 7, 1971.
[29] "The Truman Memories," *Life* XL (January 23, 1956) 104.
[30] U.S. Federal Security Agency, *The Nation's Health, A Ten-Year Program: A Report to the President* (Washington: 1948), 87.

information of that time and reflecting the emerging public policy regarding the roles of government and private efforts. In his letter of transmittal to the president, Dr. Magnuson appeared to crystalize the role of government in a manner that had never been stated so before:

> The building up of our health resources in terms of training more health personnel and providing more physical facilities must start from the ground up. We have recommended federal grants-in-aid to these and other necessary activities because we believe that the role of the federal government is to stimulate them, not to control them. Government must take the leadership in the promotion of good health; its major energies should go here rather than in extensive direct operation of health services.[31]

In other words, government should set the stage for the nation's health services—poking here, prodding there, providing information on cost and needs and assisting in financing, but generally not controlling or operating these services.[32]

As in the case of previous government commissions, there was no consensus on methods or sources of financing, but for the first time there was a consensus that voluntary health insurance might well be the means. The commission's recommendations on this point were ambiguous, but the ambiguity resulted from a willingness to place all methods on fair trial. This was new. The commission recommended that "the present prepayment plans be expanded to provide as much health service to as many people as they can . . . and be aided by government through allowing payroll deductions for government employees, removing the restrictions in organization of prepayment plans, and promoting research on health service administration." Other recommendations presaged the Medicare Act for the beneficiaries of old-age and survivors insurance enacted in 1965.

During the deliberations of the president's commission, voluntary health insurance in some form was covering 58 percent of the population of the country, compared with only 40 percent four years earlier. Then came the Eisenhower era. From 1952 to 1960, the country took a rest, as it were, from social reform stimulated by government. Voluntary health insurance had a clear field and an informal mandate to reach its natural limits without, from the

---

[31] The President's Commission on the Health Needs of the Nation, *Building America's Health: Findings and Recommendations*, 5 vols, 1952, p. vii.

[32] There is much more extensive treatment of this period in Odin W. Anderson, *The Uneasy Equilibrium; Private and Public Financing of Health Services in the United States, 1875-1965* (New Haven, Connecticut: College and University Press, 1968), p. 127-128.

viewpoint of its advocates, the constant harassment of imminent government health insurance. The more candid leaders, however, believed that such harassment was a goad to continual growth.

So voluntary health insurance stood at the beginning of a new era. When Stuart became chairman of the Blue Cross Commission in 1952, he was not sanguine. He scolded his colleagues in the manner of an Old Testament prophet. He felt the Blue Cross principles had been seriously eroded

> We found ourselves thinking and spending in insurance terms, and in some areas using the methods, technics and concepts of traditional commercial insurance. If our function is simply to provide hospital insurance to the people who wish to buy it from us in preference to buying it from long established companies with more adequate reserves, then we should rid ourselves of our responsibility to hospitals, completely abandon the service principle, eliminate the right to continuous coverage, forget about community enrollment, put more fine print in our nongroup contract, start a program of cancellation when the risk deteriorates, rate each group according to its own utilization, throw off the cloak of community service and stand for what we are: 87 relatively small companies writing hospitalization insurance.[33]

What Stuart was describing was the intensifying competition in the health insurance market. Unable to be a monopoly, Blue Cross was trimming its sails to survive without compromising its principles unduly.

[33]James E. Stuart, "Blue Cross Slips are Showing," *Modern Hospital*, August, 1953, p. 1–2. (Reprint)

Chapter Eight

The Struggle for National Accounts—The 1950s

The early 1950s witnessed a marked slowing down of the growth of Blue Cross plans. Health Services, Inc. was not as effective in facilitating the enrollment of national accounts as its organizers had hoped it would be. Private insurance companies were moving ahead of Blue Cross plans in enrollment, although the plans continued to be strong in urban areas, and especially in middle income employed groups. Although Blue Cross enrollment was slowing down, its share of the existing market was not diminishing; rather, private insurance companies were moving more rapidly into the uncovered market.

Blue Cross leaders continued to believe that the key to effective competition and continued expansion was a mechanism to enroll large national accounts. In 1955, the self-dubbed "millionaires club"—the 12 plans with at least a million members that accounted for one-half the Blue Cross total of over 51 million—assembled in an atmosphere of discreet secrecy to develop a national program of enrollment, if necessary without regard for the other 65 plans, which might be expected to drag their feet. They met in New York, where the biggest plan in the nation—Associated Hospital Service with seven million members—was located. The vehicle for this new national enrollment venture was the Blue Cross Association, not the Blue Cross Commission, thus giving the association a new and important function. According to Stuart, support for the concept within the group came quite easily.[1]

The first reference to this new function for BCA appeared in the minutes of a meeting of the Commission in Chicago on May 2, 1956. Later that month, the commission created a special Committee on Reorganization of the

---

[1] James E. Stuart, "The Blue Cross History: An Informal Biography of the Voluntary Non-Profit Prepayment Plan for Hospital Care" (Unpublished manuscript, 1966), p. 272.

National Structure as windowdressing. BCA was to be the national enrollment vehicle, and BCC was to continue its functions as a coordinating agency and trade association for approved plans, i.e., plans approved by AHA. By September 1956, 45 of the 77 plans had applied for membership in the reorganized national enrollment program. In time, all the plans became members.

Again, the Blue Cross Commission looked for a national leader who would manage the new enrollment venture with BCA as the vehicle. This time, the leader who was chosen was Basil C. MacLean, M.D. who had been associated with Blue Cross development and hospital administration since 1933. He had helped to start the New Orleans plan when he was director of the Touro Infirmary, a teaching hospital there. He was a member of the original Committee on Hospital Service started by Rorem. He was also a past president of the American Hospital Association. At the time he was asked to head the Blue Cross Association, he was commissioner of hospitals of New York City. MacLean, who was then 62, undoubtedly had the background and stature that were felt to be desirable and appropriate, but he needed competent and agressive assistants. The office was established in New York City at MacLean's request. Singsen became vice-president and treasurer, and Colman was appointed vice-president and secretary. Colman had been out of the Blue Cross field for a few years as vice-president of Johns Hopkins University, and this gave him an opportunity to return.

Their acute need was for an enrollment director, an exceedingly important post because enrollment was the objective of the association. Harold G. Pearce of the Michigan plan was "loaned" to the association—presumably for a few months, while a permanent enrollment director was sought for and recruited. Surprisingly, however, no suitable candidate was found or came forward, even at a very competitive salary.

The Blue Cross Association was a failure. Why? MacLean was an ailing man at the time, a fact not known to those who engaged him. He was a hospital consultant and continued part-time in this role. Perhaps the plans did not come forward aggressively enough with national accounts. Certainly the absence of a permanent full-time enrollment director was no help. The reason given for failure in the minutes of the Blue Cross Commission in October 1959, was: "Because there is not agreement on the basis of equalization or mutualization on national account business."[2] The fact was that the problem of

[2]Blue Cross Commission, Minutes, Chicago, October 6, 1959. Undoubtedly, Mannix, the Blue Cross gadfly of the American Blue Cross concept of 1944, was aware of the continuing difficulties of unifying Blue Cross nationally. He was not one of the 12 Blue Cross directors known as the millionaires club. He did not seem to be a team person. At the annual meeting of the American Hospital Association in New York in August 1959, Mannix

unifying Blue Cross plans for national accounts in 1956 was still beyond the capability of any one man, as it had been beyond the capability of Hawley years earlier. In the 1960s Blue Cross plans began to achieve more unity—in different circumstances and under leadership which understood the circumstances.

Blue Cross plans seemed to need a type of national account which would involve all of them simultaneously. The syndicate concept was ingenious, but not sufficient. Perhaps the first example of unified action among Blue Cross plans was the formulation of the contract with the Defense Department known as the Civilian Health and Medical Program of the Uniformed Services (CHAMPUS) in 1956. (Originally, it was called Medicare, but that name was pre-empted by the federal government and the press when health insurance for the aged became a popular political issue in the 1960s.) Through this program the Defense Department bought health services from hospitals and physicians near military installations, supplementing the official services of the Defense Department medical establishment. Initially, the contract was negotiated by the Blue Cross Commission, but administration and responsibility were transferred to the Blue Cross Association in 1956 when it was being staffed and relocated in New York City. BCA, then, became the prime contractor, and the plans became subcontractors.[3] There was no underwriting; the Defense Department paid for the services and paid the participating plans their cost of administration. Blue Cross plans in two-thirds of the states subcontracted CHAMPUS through BCA; Mutual of Omaha, a private insurance company, contracted with the Defense Department for coverage in the remaining states. Stuart wrote that "this first partnership with the government was an outstanding success."

Still, the Blue Cross Association was stumbling, and to add needed strength the purest Blue Cross protagonist in the movement was persuaded to come to New York to work with MacLean late in 1957. Stuart of the Cincinnati plan, a former chairman of the commission, took over as executive vice-president of the Blue Cross Association with the expectation that he would succeed MacLean when he retired. Stuart was then 61 years old. Like MacLean, he was regarded as a strong national leader who had enough years left to take Blue Cross

---

was invited by Dr. Edwin Crosby, executive director of the American Hospital Association, to present the American Blue Cross idea again. He had, in fact been pushing the idea for 20 years. Mannix' presentation at the AHA meeting got a great deal of publicity in the national press, led off by the *New York Times*. The audience now became a public audience, but still Mannix reported lack of enthusiasm among Blue Cross plan directors. John R. Mannix, "Prepayment, Hospitals and the Future; Needed: Strong Leadership and a Unified Blue Cross," *Hospitals*, November 1, 1959, (reprint) and personal correspondence, August 9, 1973.

[3]The Defense Department had an arrangement with the Blue Shield plans directly rather than through its association, the National Association of Blue Shield Plans.

over until younger leadership came up. Stuart's memoirs reveal that he regarded his acceptance as a last fling at making the Blue Cross idea viable nationally before he retired, although he expressed fatigue and had scolded the plans for compromising their principles five years earlier.

The internal affairs and business operations of the association continued to be headed by Singsen as vice-president and treasurer. George Heitler, an attorney and executive with 19 years of diversified experience, was recruited to serve as house counsel and assistant secretary under Colman, the association's vice-president and secretary. A beginning was made in research and public relations. To manage enrollment, Gerald M. Green was taken from Health Services, Inc.; he came as an assistant vice-president. Pearce, before he left, had set up three district enrollment offices. Restiveness with the differentiated functions—sometimes difficult to keep separate—of the Blue Cross Commission, the American Hospital Association, and Health Services, Inc. had continued.

Reporting for the Blue Cross Association at a meeting of the Blue Cross Commission in October 1959, Stuart brought up the possibility of a single national Blue Cross agency, independent of the American Hospital Association. There was a surprised reception to this concept. Many plan directors feared it meant that the Blue Cross Association was reaching for power in relation to the plans. Stuart wrote that the commission had outlived its usefulness, and the division of responsibilities between the commission and the association was too unwieldy.

Despite the seemingly unfavorable reaction, the commission and the association began to move immediately on the concept of a single agency. It was suggested, for example, that there be an exchange of representatives between the Blue Cross Association and the American Hospital Association both on their governing bodies and in their voting delegations. Further, it was proposed that the approval of Blue Cross plans should continue to be the responsibility of the American Hospital Association.

In order to make the demise of the commission as gentle as possible, the American Hospital Association took the first step by establishing a committee on the reorganization of the Blue Cross national structure. H. Charles Abbot of the Los Angeles plan and Stanley H. Saunders of Rhode Island were appointed to represent the commission. Frank Groner of Tennessee and Tol Terrell of Texas, both leaders in association affairs, represented the American Hospital Association, and William S. McNary of the Michigan plan and N. D. Helland of the Oklahoma plan represented the Blue Cross Association. Frank Groner, a well-known hospital administrator from Memphis and former president of the American Hospital Association, was appointed chairman. The committee met frequently for six months beginning in October 1959. Groner was a skillful chairman, and an agreement was achieved reaching toward the twin objectives of "strengthening Blue Cross as a national entity and toward a real partnership with the American Hospital Association.[4]

Before the annual meeting of Blue Cross plans in April 1960 in Los Angeles, specific recommendations had been formulated and accepted by the American Hospital Association, the Blue Cross Commission, and the Blue Cross Association for reassigning the functions of the commission. Again, the assistance of legal counsel was described as outstanding.[5]

The recommendations included creation of a new council on Blue Cross, prepayment, and financing by the American Hospital Association. Functions transferred to this council were: the approval program, handling of the license agreement for protection of the Blue Cross emblem, and hospital reimbursement methods. All other functions of the commission were assigned to the reorganized Blue Cross Association: (1) Inter-Plan Service Benefit Bank, (2) Inter-Plan Transfer Agreement, (3) local benefit agreement for national accounts, (4) national account agreement, and (5) national advertising program. Local plans delegated authority to the association to handle accounts with employers having employee groups in two or more states.

The partnership of the American Hospital Association and Blue Cross Association was to be visible in an interlocking board membership. AHA would have three representatives on the BCA board, and two Blue Cross representatives would be on the board of trustees of AHA.

At a meeting in April 1960, called jointly by the Blue Cross Commission and the Blue Cross Association, every plan was represented by its director and many plans by some members of their boards and senior staffs as well. Stuart recalls that it was the largest Blue Cross Commission meeting that was ever held.[6] The commission staff was given employment security either through the Blue Cross Association or the American Hospital Association's new prepayment council. Jones, the director of the abolished commission, was assigned to the staff of the council. Final approval of all these proposals was given by the house of delegates of the American Hospital Association in August 1960.

The reorganized Blue Cross Association then moved back to Chicago, and into the AHA headquarters building—another visible symbol of partnership. Stuart had become president in 1959 (MacLean died shortly

---

[4]Stuart, "The Blue Cross History," p. 295.
[5]In the forefront were Robert T. Sherman, a Chicago attorney representing the AHA and BCC, and Fred Sheffield and George Heitler of New York representing BCA. Heitler was to succeed Colman as vice-president and secretary of BCA when Colman became president of the Blue Cross plan in New York City. Heitler also continued as legal counsel.
[6]Stuart, "The Blue Cross History," p. 296.

thereafter), and his memoirs reveal understandable self-satisfaction with developments under his presidency. He had already made it known that he wished to retire not later than the spring of 1962, and after the reorganization was accomplished he devoted a great deal of his attention to finding a successor.

During the 1950s the federal government had been requested by the voluntary health insurance agencies, including Blue Cross, to provide payment by payroll deduction for its employees, as had become general for other employers. As a matter of fact, about half of all federal employees were already enrolled in Blue Cross and Blue Shield plans, with the employees paying their subscriber fees directly through group collections, without the convenience of payroll deduction. The first step the U.S. Civil Service Commission took toward provision of group insurance benefits was to enroll federal employees in group life insurance plans through a number of life insurance companies. This step led to a desire for insurance against the costs of personal health services on the part of federal employees. The Civil Service Commission and the Treasury Department first seriously considered some type of major medical or catastrophic illness coverage through private insurance companies. Blue Cross and Blue Shield representatives entered into vigorous competition, opposing this type of coverage. The Blue Cross and Blue Shield interests assumed that since private insurance companies had the life insurance contract, it was logical that Blue Cross and Blue Shield plans should get the health insurance contract.

In 1959, there appeared to be support in the Congress for some type of federal contributory scheme. Hearings were held on two bills, and, finally, Public Law 86–382 was approved in September 1959, to become effective July 1, 1960. Representatives from all the major health insurance agencies had given testimony. The Civil Service Commission was then empowered to develop a health insurance program for federal employees, providing for options among existing health insurance alternatives, and between two benefit options called high and low options. The federal government contributed half the cost of the low benefit option. If the employee wanted the high option he had to pay the extra cost himself. Even so, the employees overwhelmingly selected the high option.

A joint Blue Cross and Blue Shield committee was set up by the national associations—one instance in which there was a wholehearted common endeavor between the two bodies. Blue Cross was represented by Stuart, F. P. Rawlings of the Washington, D.C. plan, and J. Douglas Colman, who was then vice-president and secretary of the Blue Cross Association, which was still in New York and had not yet been superseded the Blue Cross Commission. Blue Shield was represented by John Castellucci, who at that time was director of the National Association of Blue Shield Plans, Donald Stubbs, M.D., president of the

Washington, D.C., Blue Shield plan and a long-time leader in Blue Shield, and Don Diller of Pennsylvania. The national enrollment agencies, Health Insurance, Inc. of Blue Cross and Medical Indemnity of America for Blue Shield, were also involved.

The joint committee found itself in the position of having to speak for all member plans in Blue Cross and Blue Shield, but without specific authority. There simply was not time to clear everything with member plans as negotiations with the Civil Service Commission proceeded. Stuart wrote, for example, "The committee had the courage to commit the member plans with the Civil Service Commission to courses of action which it fervently hoped the plans would accede to, and was greatly relieved when most of them eventually did so."[7] Of course, it would have been foolish for the plans to reject three million new members for the sake of local autonomy. The federal employees program helped to unify Blue Cross plans. Blue Shield plans were even less coordinated than Blue Cross, and Castellucci observed that the federal employee contract also helped to unify Blue Shield: "Every time we wanted to make a little change up to this time we would have to go to all the plans, but with the federal employees contract we just announced it and sat back and waited for the noise, but none came."[8]

On the Blue Cross side great credit was given to J. Douglas Colman for being the spokesman to Congress during preparation of the bill and in the hearings. He was assisted by Edwin R. Werner of the National Association of Blue Shield Plans. As noted, both Blue Cross and Blue Shield plans accepted the final arrangement made by their Washington representatives, who may have exceeded their charge.

Blue Cross now had a nationwide pattern of benefits, a method of rating which all the plans except one eventually approved. The single exception was the Cleveland plan, which serviced the claims locally, with underwriting done by Cincinnati. Even before the Blue Cross Association became the sole national agency for Blue Cross plans its success in obtaining the federal employees contract enhanced it as a national agency. The Federal Employees Health Benefit Program got off to a good start in 1960 and has, by all reasonable standards, been a successful operation from the standpoint of all parties:[9] the various prepayment and insurance agencies, the employees, the providers, and the Civil Service Commission.

[7]Ibid, p. 284.
[8]Interview in Ft. Lauderdale, March 23, 1973.
[9]Odin W. Anderson and J. Joel May, *The Federal Employees Health Benefits Program: 1961–1968; A Model For National Health Insurance?* Perspectives A9 (Chicago: Center for Health Administration Studies, University of Chicago, 1971).

Chapter Nine

Local Strengths and Difficulties

Obviously, unless Blue Cross plans had established a solid working base in each state, prospects for a strong federation of plans cooperating for national accounts and national purposes would never have been possible. This account may have given the impression that the only wheeling and dealing worth chronicling was on the national level, and it is this level that constitutes the major portion of the Blue Cross story. The seeming emphasis on the national picture stems from the objective of this study: to show the struggle of the Blue Cross idea to become a national entity in an economy dominated by large corporations having large groups of employees in many different localities throughout the country. Without viable local bases joined to a viable national agency, Blue Cross plans would be unable to play a strong role in the national health economy, and, in fact, the local plans themselves would be weaker. Thus detailed attention to the creation and development of local plans one by one as they came into existence and grew throughout these early decades would not especially serve the purpose of this particular study—interesting though such a story would certainly be. However, it does seem to be necessary here to give some insight into local problems encountered in some parts of the country. If these had not been resolved at some level of accommodation, they would have hindered operations unduly, and perhaps destroyed the plans. Few of these difficult situations are in the record with any more than passing mention, and the isolated facts in the reports are too stark for accurate interpretation. The accounts here have been gathered mainly from interviews.

No Blue Cross plan was permitted to go bankrupt. The plans in the early days were like hospitals, and perhaps churches—they were not allowed to die. A bankrupt Blue Cross plan would reflect on the movement. Plans that had financial difficulties seemed to lack competent leadership and had insufficient hospital or medical backing. New Mexico[1] in the fifties and Montana[2] later are examples. The usual solution was to merge with another plan.

There were also some jurisdictional problems. Blue Cross plans were not supposed to overlap service territories, but there were exceptions—tolerated by the national Blue Cross agency for lack of power to insist on change. North Carolina was the outstanding example, with plans based at Chapel Hill and Durham, each headed by a capable executive well known in the state. The rivalry was fierce at times, and even Hawley, during his short tenure as director of the national Blue Cross agency, did not succeed in merging them when he visited North Carolina as an arbitration emissary. E. B. Crawford of the Chapel Hill plan said: "It was called an original sin that they couldn't get rid of for years."[3] The merger was brought about, finally, when the two executives reached retirement age at about the same time. A problem of overlapping jurisdictions still remains in Illinois, between the Rockford plan and the Chicago-based plan that covers the rest of the state.[4]

The most bothersome problems, however, stemmed from conflicts between Blue Cross plans and medical societies. The promotion of a single hospital and medical package backed by the respective providers had obvious administrative advantages. There were bitter struggles in southern California, Louisiana, Wisconsin, Minnesota, Oregon, Montana, Washington, and New Mexico. The Los Angeles Blue Cross plan and California Physicians' Service (Blue Shield) ceased to cooperate in 1950, for example, and Blue Cross wrote physicians' services and Blue Shield hospital coverage on an indemnity basis.[5]

In the state of Washington, where country medical society–sponsored medical service plans started in the 1930s, the plans also wrote hospital insurance. The hospitals complained of low indemnities for patients covered by the county society plans, and Washington Blue Cross was established in 1942. It also covered physicians' services. From that time until 1970 there were chronic conflicts between the county medical society plans and the Blue Cross plan. As related by C. J. Kretchmer: "They are direct competitors, the county society plans being contracting agents for doctors selling hospitalization indemnity and Blue Cross being a contracting agency with hospitals selling indemnity for physicians' services."[6]

[1] As reported by Reginald Cahalane, Walpole, New Hampshire, on August 5, 1971. He was sent as a consultant to New Mexico to revive a foundering plan. At that time, he was on the staff of the Blue Cross Commission as field representative.

[2] As reported by William Guy, Los Angeles, April 25, 1973, who accepted the challenge of getting the Montana plan on its feet.

[3] Interview with E. B. Crawford, Chapel Hill, North Carolina, May 21, 1971.

[4] Interview with Kenneth Clark, Rockford, Illinois, December 19, 1972.

[5] Interview with Charles Abbott, Los Angeles, April 25, 1973.

[6] Interview with C. J. Kretchmer in Seattle, Washington, May 1, 1971.

In the 1960s in Minnesota there were many conflicts between the Blue Cross and Blue Shield plans, seesawing between Blue Cross selling physicians' services on an indemnity basis and Blue Shield selling hospital care at times, to joint promotion of hospital and medical benefits at other times. In 1970 the Blue Shield plan was virtually bankrupt, and the state insurance commissioner moved in. Blue Shield made an appeal to Blue Cross to bail it out, which was done in a few days, and the two organizations became a joint operation. Later, they merged. Abbot Lee Fletcher, the Blue Cross legal counsel and long-time board member, wrote: "The assumption by Blue Cross of these management duties and the guarantee to Blue Shield contract holders certainly rank as one of the most graphic illustrations of the underlying and unselfish concerns of Minnesota Blue Cross for the welfare of the people of the state of Minnesota."[7]

Another example is in Wisconsin, where a complicated situation developed between rival medical factions centered in Madison and Milwaukee, with the Milwaukee-based Blue Cross plan caught in between. Milwaukee Blue Cross cooperated with the Milwaukee Blue Shield plan on hospital and medical benefits. The Madison-based Blue Shield plan wanted to be the statewide physicians' plan and added hospital service to its benefits. A merger between the Madison and Milwaukee medical plans is eminently logical but has not taken place, though there are indications that hostility has lessened considerably.[8]

The degree to which difficulties between Blue Cross plans and medical societies interfered with the pace and extent of Blue Cross growth is not easy to measure. Certainly they can be regarded as hindrances to overall development and forward movement. There were many instances of cooperation between Blue Cross and Blue Shield plans, the pivotal plans in Michigan and the auto industry being a case in point. The most common corporate and administrative structure of Blue Cross and Blue Shield plans is two corporations and two chief executives, though less than half the plans are still so organized. Plans with this structure are mainly in the East and Middle West, and they represent the dominant pattern in terms of their enrollment and urban bases.

The next most common form, with about one-quarter of the plans, is two corporations and boards, with one chief executive. These are smaller plans scattered all over the country, with the significant exception of the large Illinois plan in Chicago. There are fewer than a dozen plans with one corporation offering both hospital and physician services. These are also rather scattered and

---

[7] Abbott Lee Fletcher, *History of Minnesota Blue Cross* (No publisher and no date), and interview in Minneapolis, August 2, 1972.

[8] The details of this conflict are candidly documented in Frank Sinclair, *Blue Cross in Wisconsin* (Milwaukee: Blue Cross, 1965); also interviews with Leo E. Suycott, Milwaukee, August 9, 1972, and Charles H. Crownhart, Madison, August 10, 1972.

relatively small.[9] The remaining plans do not coordinate with Blue Shield at all. These are mainly on the West Coast and in Louisiana.

It would seem to be a reasonable conclusion that if Blue Shield plans had been wholeheartedly supported by the American Medical Association and the local medical societies and in turn had joined forces with Blue Cross plans for joint hospital and physicians' service prepayment they could have dominated voluntary health insurance. It is unlikely that they would have had a monopoly, but they could have become a strong, unified professional reference point.

A final and important observation should be made regarding human resources and interests. There have been and still are many citizens who contributed greatly to Blue Cross plans as public members of the local boards. Three of them have been granted the Justin Ford Kimball Award for distinguished service to the Blue Cross idea over the years. They were George A. Newbury, Buffalo, New York, a banker; John Paynter, Detroit, a business man; and Herman Somers, Princeton, New Jersey, a professor.[10] All these and many others represent the reservoir of public-spirited talent willing to contribute without remuneration to public service programs. People with such talent and interest constitute a resource that has been characteristic of American Society.

---

[9] A recent development in New York City may well influence the restructuring of Blue Cross and Blue Shield plan relationships for the future. The Associated Hospital Service and the Blue Shield plan of New York City formed one corporation in February 1974. Interview with Edwin R. Werner, February 27, 1974.

[10] Others who should be mentioned are: Fred Wardenburg, Wilmington, Delaware, of the duPont Company; George Putnam, Boston, investment banker; Marion Folsom, Rochester, New York, one-time secretary of the Department of Health, Education and Welfare; John Manion, Chicago, banker; Kenneth D. MacCall, Providence, Rhode Island, businessman; George Watts Hill, Durham, North Carolina; Albert Koorie, New Orleans; Abbott Fletcher, Minneapolis, lawyer; William Gosnell, Rochester, New York; Harry B. Kennedy, New Haven; Thomas Gates, Jr., Philadelphia, one-time secretary of the Navy; Phillips M. Payson, Portland, Maine; Forrest F. Dodds, Kansas City, Missouri; William E. Lingelbock, Jr., Philadelphia; Orville H. Bullitt, Philadelphia; Thomas C. Boushall, Richmond, Virginia.

Chapter Ten

Toward National Capability—
The 1960s Into the 1970s

When the Blue Cross Association became the sole national entity as a federation of Blue Cross plans in 1960, its potential, if not actual, strength was the possibility that it could achieve operation as a unified local and national program. Together with Blue Shield plans for physicians' services, the membership base was sizable, although it was no longer growing in relation to private insurance companies. More than 30 percent of the population, i.e., 56 million or so, was enrolled in Blue Cross–Blue Shield plans, no mean base from which to thrust further in expansion of benefits, improvements in member services, and strengthening of relationship with providers. Private insurance comapnies were extremely competitive, having made both relative and absolute gains since the early fifties. Competitively and as a national factor in health services financing, the Blue Cross and Blue Shield plans probably had more influence than private insurance companies—partly because the several hundred insurance companies in the business made concerted action difficult. Blue Cross and Blue Shield plans were the single largest unified entity for national accounts. Only the larger private insurance companies could compete effectively in this arena. By 1963, of all persons with some hospital insurance, 54 percent had some private insurance hospital coverage. Forty-six percent had some Blue Cross coverage.[1] The main enrollment strength of Blue Cross plans lay in the metropolitan areas, where Blue Cross had 52 percent of the population. In other rural but nonfarm areas, Blue Cross had 45 percent, and 36 percent of the rural farm population was enrolled in Blue Cross plans. Private insurance companies had comparable and

[1] Figures from Ronald Anderson and Odin W. Anderson, *A Decade of Health Services; Social Survey Trends in Use and Expenditures* (Chicago: University of Chicago Press, 1960), 85.

81

Table 10–1. Percent of Households Covered by Hospital Insurance in 1963

Residence	Blue Cross	Private Insurance
Urban	52	57
Rural nonfarm	45	56
Rural farm	36	68

somewhat larger enrollments in all three types of residential areas, but particularly in rural farm areas (see Table 10–1).

The comparative success of private insurance companies in rural areas was due to sales and underwriting methods not used by Blue Cross plans. Private insurance companies had extensive agency systems promoting sales of health insurance to individuals instead of only groups, along with other types of insurance such as life and casualty. Inherently high costs of selling to individuals necessitated benefits that were low in relation to hospital costs in order to keep the premiums at an attractively low level. Blue Cross plan benefits and prices were based directly on going hospital costs. During the fifties, many Blue Cross plans experimented with various types of individual enrollment techniques in order to reach self-employed people, such as farmers. They carried individual enrollment as far as it was possible to do and still maintain the low costs associated with group enrollment.[2] The self-employed and those in small business establishments continue to be a difficult segment of the population to cover. Even in proposals for universal health insurance they are handled as a special category.

A favorite and easy measure of health insurance performance is the portion of the hospital bill paid by a particular insuring agency. Blue Cross plans were clearly paying a higher portion of the hospital bill in group contracts than the private insurance companies were. In 1963, Blue Cross in 73 percent of all its admissions was paying 90 percent or more of the bill, compared with 59 percent for private insurance companies. For nongroup enrollment admissions, Blue Cross was slightly ahead of private insurance companies in paying 90 percent of the bill, 35 and 32 percent respectively.[3] Blue Shield plans paid 90 percent or more of the surgical fee in 52 percent of admissions, while private insurance companies paid 90 percent or more in 41 percent of the cases.[4] It is also

[2]See Sol Levine, Odin W. Anderson, and Gerald Gordon, *Non-Group Enrollment for Health Insurance; A Study of Administrative Approaches of Blue Cross Plans* (Cambridge, Massachusetts: Harvard University Press, 1957).

[3]Ronald Andersen and Odin W. Anderson, *A Decade of Health Services: Social Survey Trends in Use and Expenditures* (Chicago: University of Chicago Press, 1960, p. 107.

[4]Ibid, p. 104.

significant that Blue Cross patients were more likely to be in hospital accommodations classed as expensive than were patients insured with private insurance companies, 51 and 37 percent respectively.[5] In terms of benefits, Blue Cross was relatively more attractive.

Although Blue Cross plans had a smaller proportion of the total market than private insurance companies, it would seem that it was stronger than the numerical proportion would indicate because of its firmer anchorage in large metropolitan areas, its relatively favorable performance in paying hospital bills, its contractual relationship with hospitals, its national accounts with industrial giants such as General Motors, Ford, Chrysler, and U.S. Steel, and the interplan agreements for benefit and membership transfers. In addition, CHAMPUS and federal employee contracts helped to stabilize the national association through the means of common objectives. The private insurance companies had no comparable central agency through which they cooperated in the manner of the Blue Cross Association among its member plans. In contrast, in fact, the private insurance companies were competitive among themselves.

Such were the circumstances when the Blue Cross Association was reorganized under Stuart. As the association began to look for a successor to Stuart, the high stakes were the strengthening and furtherance of a unified Blue Cross system. Familiar names among Blue Cross plan directors were mentioned as successors. Emphasis was now placed on youth; presumably the successful candidate would be under 50. Blue Cross was felt to be mature enough so as not to require older statesmen. An apparently open-ended future required a leader who was young enough to live into the future and help to shape it. In addition, someone had to be found who was not associated with past prejudices and vested interests among plan directors. Instead, an outsider was sought. Long-range continuity of leadership was now needed.

This leadership was found. Surprisingly, a search committee of the Blue Cross Association began to look at the people in the universities who were directing programs in hospital and health service administration. These programs had burgeoned to a status of prominence, and the field of hospital administration was rapidly being professionalized. Two directors of university programs were being scouted by BCA, according to Stuart: Ray Trussell, M.D., director of the program in hospital and health administration, School of Public Health and Medical Administration, Columbia University; and Walter J. McNerney, director of the program in hospital administration at the Graduate School of Business of the University of Michigan. Trussell, senior to McNerney by 10 years (McNerney was in his mid-thirties), reportedly was not interested.

McNerney was completing a massive study of the total health service

[5] Ibid, p. 103.

situation in the state of Michigan, supported by a generous grant from the Kellogg Foundation. The study was inaugurated because Blue Cross of Michigan had requested approval of a rate increase of more than 20 percent by the State Department of Insurance. The upshot was the creation of an independent study commission, staffed by McNerney from his academic base. This study gave McNerney great prominence, both in Michigan and nationally, because of its scope, public policy importance, and the bellwether nature of Michigan itself, which had pioneered in Blue Cross and Blue Shield development and in the field of public health generally.[6] McNary of the Michigan Blue Cross plan was able to watch McNerney at close range. He liked what he saw and he was empowered to offer McNerney the presidency of BCA.

There is no indication that McNerney hesitated. His rise in the academic world had been rapid, and his entrance into the world of action was almost a quantum leap, considering the national base which the Blue Cross venture had now as Stuart was leaving. It is remarkable that the Blue Cross directors were willing to have a leader who was younger than any of them, and an academician as well. It might be said uncharitably that this indicated the depth of their desperation; a more valid view, it would seem, was their prescience and sense of risk-taking. True, the Blue Cross directors had relatively secure posts, personally, in their local plans, but commitments were still being made to create a manipulable and cohesive system which could function simultaneously on national, regional, and local levels.

That McNerney saw this challenge immediately was evident in his actions as soon as he accepted the offer. One move he made at once was to ask for a 100 percent increase in the dues paid by member plans. This was granted. In short order, he began then to assemble a staff that could act more effectively than had been done previously to provide information and service to the plans and national contracts.[7] In time, a committee was established, headed by Fritz Lattner of the Des Moines, Iowa, plan, now retired, to formulate performance indicators by which plan performance could be monitored and evaluated. If Blue Cross plans were going to operate through the Blue Cross Association on national contracts, the association needed to measure the performance capabilities of the member plans with which it would subcontract.

While strengthening the national operating base of the Blue Cross

[6]Walter J. McNerney and Study Staff. *Hospital and Medical Economics: A Study of Population, Services, Costs, Methods of Payment, and Controls.* 2 vols. (Chicago: Hospital Research and Educational Trust, 1962).

[7]Throughout his tenure as BCA president, McNerney has expanded the staff repeatedly to accommodate new functions. In 1969, he hired D. Eugene Sibery as executive vice-president. Sibery, a hospital administrator who became an executive of Michigan Blue Cross and later, the Greater Detroit hospital planning agency, devoted the greater part of his time to BCA operations so McNerney was able to give more attention to relations with the plans, government, business and labor groups, and the public.

system, McNerney began to move into the problem of hospital and medical services for the aged, which had become an intense political issue. Given the past policy positions of the American Hospital Association, the American Medical Association, and a consortium of private insurance companies through the Health Insurance Association of America regarding government health insurance, the Blue Cross Association was in the middle of an explosive situation in relation to its peers. The standard position of these provider and payer agencies was in favor of government subsidy of health services for the poor, and one method to implement this subsidy was for the government to enroll low income people in voluntary health insurance plans. This was already being done in a number of states.

The aged, however, did not fit neatly into the poor category, even though two-thirds of those over age 65 had incomes at or under what was regarded as the poverty level, and the majority were no longer considered as part of the labor market. Furthermore, they were high users of health services by virtue of their age, disabilities, and illnesses and therefore were already a disproportionate drain on the pooled funds of the prepayment and insurance agencies. The rate structure needed a loading factor for the aged enrollees who were either still in the labor force or had left employment and continued coverage under individual arrangements. Loading of rates for the aged was becoming common among insurance agencies, and the need to increase rates to cover the costs of aged enrollees was a burden to all insuring agencies, including Blue Cross plans. Insurance companies and Blue Cross plans had tried various methods of covering the aged after they left employment. In short, voluntary health insurance was inherently incapable of sharing a high risk equitably among its various components unless there was agreement to build the aged into the rate structure. The competition was too great among the private insurance companies, and competition was always a factor between Blue Cross plans and insurance companies. Under the circumstances, Blue Cross actions regarding the aged would seem to have gone as far as was feasible by providing mechanisms for conversion on termination of employment and open enrollment. Another problem was the resistance of both employees and employers to the increased payroll deductions for higher rates needed to cover growing numbers of aged. In short, medical care for the aged was becoming felt as a broad, middle income burden which should properly be shifted to the public sector.

McNerney approached health insurance for the aged frontally by setting up a study committee jointly with the Blue Cross Association and the American Hospital Association to assemble data on income and health problems of the aged and ponder the implications of the data.[8] Early in 1962, there was a

---

[8] Blue Cross Association and American Hospital Association, Joint Committee, *Financing Health Care of the Aged*, pts. I and II (Chicago: 1962).

joint meeting of the member plans of the Blue Cross Association and the house of delegates of the American Hospital Association. Present also were representatives of the American Medical Association and Blue Shield.[9] Frank Groner, president of the American Hospital Association, and Stuart, chairman of the Blue Cross Association, presided jointly. McNerney was then president. Dr. Edwin L. Crosby, executive vice-president of AHA, and McNerney presented the factual background and the problem.

A joint resolution resulted which accepted the need for government assistance in providing hospital care for the aged, but the participants did not reach agreement on a governmental program for all the aged through the Social Security payroll tax mechanism. Instead, the resolution read that the particular source of funds was not the affair of the hospitals or Blue Cross plans and urged that government subsidize the aged through Blue Cross on the basis of a simple incomes test involving a short report form. A forthright stand in favor of the Social Security mechanism would have been indiscreet; the medical profession could not be alienated unduly, because hospitals have to live with physicians every day.

The events leading to enactment of the Medicare amendments to the Social Security Act in 1965 hardly need to be documented here. There are several accounts of the politics and the convergence of political forces and interests that resulted finally in the combined coverage of both hospital and physicians services.[10] The aged as a group had proved to be inconveniently ambiguous politically; they were not all poor, they were expensive to insure, and thus they became a cutting edge of public policy once their income levels were ignored. The United States entered universal health insurance through an age group.

The United States also entered universal health insurance through an intermediary mechanism for payment to the providers. There were already precedents: CHAMPUS, the federal employees, and enrollment of the indigent in voluntary health insurance plans. Whenever government is given a mandate and a responsibility to act quickly to provide health care for millions of people, it has

[9]James E. Stuart, "The Blue Cross History: An Informal Biography of the Voluntary Non-Profit Prepayment Plan for Hospital Care" (Unpublished manuscript, 1966), p. 313.

[10]In addition to Odin W. Anderson *The Uneasy Equilibrium; Private and Public Financing of Health Services in the United States, 1875–1965* (New Haven, Connecticut: College and University Press, 1968), there are James L. Sundquist, *Politics and Policy: The Eisenhower, Kennedy and Johnson Years* (Washington, D.C.: Brookings Institution, 1968), chap. VII; Max J. Skidmore, *Medicare and the American Rhetoric of Reconciliation* (University, Alabama: University of Alabama Press, 1970); Herman M. Somers and Anne R. Somers, *Medicare and the Hospitals; Issues and Prospects* (Washington, D.C.: Brookings Institution, 1967); Theodore R. Marmor with Jan S. Marmor, *The Politics of Medicare* (London, England: Routledge and Kegan Paul, 1970).

turned to the private health sector. In the Medicare Act, Congress authorized the use of private intermediaries. When it became apparent to the prepayment and insurance agencies that Medicare in some form was imminent, they then sought some sort of intermediary role in order to remain in the stream. The Blue Cross Association under McNerney's leadership moved quickly to espouse the intermediary role, although there was resistance among a few Blue Cross plans. The addition of 19 million people 65 years of age and over, including the four to five million already enrolled, with only a year to tool up, was staggering to contemplate and undertake.

When Medicare was enacted, about two-thirds of the people 65 years of age and over, or approximately 13 million, had some form of health insurance. Significantly, 70 percent of these were enrolled in nongroup contracts, a type of coverage which was not as good as group contracts.[11] The 13 million aged with some coverage were to be shifted from Blue Cross and Blue Shield plans and private insurance companies to Medicare. Many of those already covered, however, continued their coverage in the private sector as a supplement to the benefits in Medicare. The private sector, and particularly Blue Cross and Blue Shield plans, made special efforts toward that end. Aside from the public service aspects, Medicare made it easier for the private sector to write supplemental benefits and continue the direct relationship with these subscribers.

The Blue Cross Association–Social Security Administration relationship was formalized by a prime contract between the two parties. The Association in turn subcontracted with its member Blue Cross plans, which contracted with their member hospitals. Blue Cross Association as prime contractor is responsible for the fiscal soundness and general performance of member plans. The government pays the association a management fee. Blue Cross is not an underwriter; the Social Security Administration is the underwriter.

Congress intended that intermediaries should be used. Why? Was the decision based on an ideological concept of the role of government in the health service economy? Did Congress not wish to enlarge the federal bureaucracy? Or did it wish to ensure the preservation of the private health insurance industry? Or, with no time to consider these underlying values shaping public policy, did the Congress simply do the expedient thing by using the private sector, which already had the staff and machinery to pay hospital and medical bills? Or, finally, did Congress feel that the providers would not cooperate unless their chosen intermediaries were used? This last is the prevailing view. As with all public policy issues and their eventual resolution, however, the particular

[11] Andersen and Anderson, p. 88.

outcome probably did not spring from a single motive, but from several. Undoubtedly, speed and the existence of ready machinery were important and very likely the precipitating factors, along with the pressure from providers. So far, the Congress has shown no desire to have the government either run or jeopardize the enterprises that are already in existence.

The Blue Cross Association moved quickly to the heart of this public policy problem—how to implement Medicare—and became the prime contractor for over 90 percent of the Medicare expenditures for hospital service.

The task of taking on 90 percent of Medicare for hospital service was a trying one, but it was a prime factor in strengthening Blue Cross unity and capability to achieve a common objective. To some extent, current business had to be neglected in order to tool up for Medicare, but Blue Cross plans succeeded in setting up the administrative machinery and facilitating cash flow to hospitals from Medicare. McNerney took personal control over negotiating the prime contract and establishing the administrative machinery for the first two years, with the assistance of Singsen. Obviously, the stakes were extremely high. Thereafter, Blue Cross hired an administrative vice-president, Bernard Tresnowski, a hospital administrator from Michigan, to head up Medicare prime contract administration and negotiations.

The decade of the 1960s was a very busy and complicated period for the Blue Cross system. Complications were increasing because of the changing nature of hospitals and medical care, the entrance of government into the provision of care, and rising consumer expectations.[12] This was the decade when questions were raised more insistently and seriously than ever regarding the legitimacy of contemporary institutions, both private and public. Were they operating in the public interest, or purely for private and special privilege interests? In the case of hospital service and its rising cost, were Blue Cross and the hospitals in collusion against the public? The constant tension as to whom Blue Cross represented, the public or the hospitals, was raised to higher intensity. The Blue Cross Association and the member plans preferred to believe that they were operating mainly as public and community agencies helping to pay hospital bills and were not simply a financial conduit for hospitals. Questions were raised about the relationship of the Blue Cross Association and the American Hospital Association on the national level, and the heavy hospital representation on the boards of some Blue Cross plans. Was this not a conflict of interest? As long ago as 1946, Rorem had tried to clarify this difficult problem

---

[12]In an interview with Fritz Lattner in Des Moines, December 6, 1972, I asked if he would do it over again. *Lattner*: "Yes, but not at this time. If something was wrong [in the early days] we could do something about it. In Medicare now, for example, we must turn to someone else [government] if something is wrong."

in his testimony before the U.S. Senate Committee on Education and Labor on a government health insurance bill: "On the one hand the Blue Cross plan represents the public as consumers. On the other hand, the hospitals represent the public as producers. So the Blue Cross is a link between the hospitals which produce the care and the consumers who receive it."[13]

In this context, there were discussions about separation of the Blue Cross Association and the American Hospital Association. The spirit and content of these discussions are reflected in a joint memorandum of March 31, 1971, from McNerney of the Blue Cross Association and Crosby of the American Hospital Association to the joint committee of the two associations regarding their organizational and operational relationships. Initiated by the Blue Cross Association, the memorandum reviewed how relations between Blue Cross plans and hospitals had been influenced by these considerations:

1. Hospital need for reasonably predictable income in a context of weak government financing program, spotty self-payment, and slowly evolving insurance company interest. This need embraced patient care, education, research, and community medicine.
2. Consumer need for service at the time of illness, as opposed to cash indemnity, and associated values of freedom from cancellation and ability to transfer benefits.
3. The practical requirements of a contract between Blue Cross and hospitals to assure provider guarantee of service.
4. Need for mutual support of a nonprofit, community ethic in the face of many adversary forces, including the professions.
5. Widespread public concern with availability of hospital beds and primary focus on the acute medical episode.

The memorandum pointed out that although some of the same conditions had continued, others were significantly different:

1. Disinclination of hospitals to guarantee service with viable financing alternative available, and interest in full reimbursement from all service.
2. Greater accent on primary care, i.e., a wide variety of benefits beyond hospital care, such as drugs and dental services.
3. Greater accent on corporate accountability energized by two major blocs, voters and consumers, with the following implications.
   (a) Greater government control over aspects of corporate activity unregu-

[13]Blue Cross Commission "Self-Portrait," 1946, p. 14.

lated by government, such as the composition of boards of directors.
(b) Concern over conflicts of interest.
(c) Need to strengthen various channels of consumer influence, e.g.,
hospital boards, Blue Cross boards, public adversary committees, and
the electorate. All are needed to counterbalance the strong (and
understandable) forces of institutionalization.
(d) Consumer wariness of good intentions, no matter how professional, as a
major way to balance consumer-provider interests; the honest adversary
is seen as a more dependable way for the future.

The honest adversary is a key concept in interest group politics and a
pluralistic political system. McNerney invokes it often. The Blue Cross
Association was seeking from its member plans more room to maneuver
unilaterally at national and local levels in its attempt to absorb and balance off
the forces at work. McNerney wanted to be freer to represent both the public
and the hospitals simultaneously and with differential intensities depending on
the circumstances, in one instance taking the side of the public and in another
instance the side of the hospitals.

Perhaps the tight wire act that Blue Cross was engaged in at the time
of the joint memorandum was discernible in McNerney's annual report to the
membership in April 1971. He described provider attitudes:

> All are seeking greater reimbursement. There is no unanimity
> regarding solutions to major problems. Old loyalties are being tested.
> A common theme for each is keeping or reaching the center of the
> stage. A professional weighing of political, economic, and health
> components, and a quest for a common middle ground are unlikely.
> The political pressures and threats of national health insurance have
> to date served to exacerbate old tensions, e.g., doctor and hospital,
> rather than heal them. Sensing this, the consumer wants more and
> more to know where Blue Cross stands and as whose representative.
> Importantly, providers need leadership . . . a rallying point pointed
> to health, not illness or the requirements of professionalism . . . and
> we must step up to that challenge, not by uncritically serving built-in
> interests, but by leadership.

These observations were made at the time events were taking place
in Pennsylvania shaping the future relationships of Pennsylvania Blue Cross plans
and hospitals. In January 1971 a new insurance commissioner was appointed in
Pennsylvania, Herbert S. Denenberg. Shortly thereafter, the Greater Philadelphia
Blue Cross plan applied for a rate increase of 43 percent, and the other Blue
Cross plans in Pennsylvania were to do the same. In Rorem's estimation, the

most important feature of the Philadelphia Blue Cross negotiations with the insurance commissioner was the direct confrontation of the Department of Insurance and the Delaware Valley Hospital Council, because in previous negotiations about subscriber rates most of the discussions had occurred between Blue Cross and the Hospital Council.[14] The Insurance commissioner had played mainly the role of arbitrator on facts and issues placed before the public officials.

Even so, there was a precedent in Pennsylvania for insurance commissioner intervention, although not in the depth and scope of the Denenberg action. In 1958, the then commissioner of insurance, Francis R. Smith, was alarmed at the requests for rather large rate increases from three Blue Cross plans in Pennsylvania. Smith was sympathetic to the Blue Cross concept (as is Denenberg) and feared that the plans would become bankrupt in the face of steadily rising hospital costs unless stiff rate increases were approved. The familiar recommendations were joint purchasing among hospitals, elimination of unnecessary duplication of facilities and services, and increased subscriber representation on the Blue Cross boards.[15] In addition, Commissioner Smith had exhorted the Blue Cross plans and hospitals: "Contrary to the expressed views of certain hospital witnesses appearing at the hearings [on rates], I believe that there must be genuine bargaining between the Blue Cross organizations and the hospitals on an arms-length basis, in working out hospital reimbursement contracts."[16]

However, as Denenberg discovered, the commissioner was charged by law to approve both the rates to Blue Cross subscribers and the payments made to hospitals contracting with Blue Cross. Denenberg denied the Blue Cross request pending review of the Insurance Department's control over the rates paid to hospitals. He did not challenge the accuracy of the statistical and financial data. Rorem observed that it seemed apparent to the commissioner that Blue Cross needed more money to reimburse hospitals at reasonable rates during a period of rising prices, increasing wages, and higher costs of construction. The commissioner directed his attention largely to subscriber demands, hospital management, and community requirements. Instead of Blue Cross being on trial for charging too much for hospital care protection, the institutions came under criticism for not giving subscribers their money's worth. This led the commissioner to also consider broad questions of health administration and finance. To this end the Delaware Valley Hospital Council received from the

[14]The substance of this case is taken from C. Rufus Rorem, "The New Philadelphia Blue Cross Hospital Agreement; Milestone or Millstone?" (Unpublished, 1973).
[15]Abstract of the adjudications of Pennsylvania Insurance Commissioner Francis R. Smith, in *Hospitals* 32 (May 16, 1958): 101+.
[16]Ibid, p. 122.

Insurance Department a list of 95 questions relating to the methods and nature of reimbursement of hospitals by the Philadelphia Blue Cross plan plus other matters such as utilization review, disclosure, malpractice review, limitations on programs and expenditures, subscriber contract, hospital economics, and consumer representation.

During the hearings, according to Rorem, the commissioner assumed the posture of a representative of the public (at least the subscribers). Blue Cross was advised by the commissioner to take the initiative in appraising hospital costs, quality, and efficiency, and to concern itself with both operating and capital expenses. Without going into unnecessary details of the agreement between Blue Cross and hospitals, it placed Blue Cross and hospitals in postures of mutual concern for the public welfare.

As Rorem described it: "The agreement places Blue Cross in the role of an agency representing and protecting the interests of millions of subscribers in their search for adequate health care. The hospitals, in turn, accept responsibility for effective use of the personnel and facilities available within their walls or under their control." Rorem is sage enough to observe that "the Philadelphia experience did not 'settle' anything. But it did bring to public attention some important aspects of health service financing which had been considered primarily the province of providers of health care [hospitals, practitioners] and the large scale group payment agencies, private and public."

The rate increase was granted. The Philadelphia Blue Cross experience helped to direct attention to the delivery problems themselves, to the problem of management, and not solely Blue Cross and hospital reimbursement negotiations. Although some action was taken in this direction, the concept itself was not particularly new. The problem of influencing the entire delivery system was seriously addressed in McNerney's two volume study in Michigan.

In the Pennsylvania context, McNerney justified this Blue Cross role in a statement before the Senate Subcommittee on Anti-Trust and Monopoly, on January 28, 1971:

> The roots of Blue Cross plans are in the communities and areas they serve. Evidence of this is seen in the hundreds of community representatives serving on Blue Cross boards without pay or reward of any kind, devoting many hours each month to development of policies, solution of problems and the adaptation of Blue Cross services to emerging social needs.[17]

To document this assertion: he reported that in 1970 there were

[17]A statement concerning the high cost of hospitalization, prepared for the Subcommittee on Anti-Trust and Monopoly, U.S. Senate, January 28, 1971, p. 2.

1,877 members on Blue Cross boards of directors nationwide. They were classified as follows: 44 percent public; 24 percent executives of health institutions; 18 percent public trustees of health institutions; and 14 percent from the medical profession. He observed that if hospital trustees who are not health professionals are regarded as public representatives, 62 percent of the Blue Cross plan board members then represent the public and the number is increasing[18] The key element in the Blue Cross edifice is the contract with the hospitals. The contract spells out the details of mutual accountability. It not only guarantees the service, but also specifies the method and basis of payment by each plan for the care of its subscribers.

In 1971, 74 million people, or 36 percent of the population, were enrolled in Blue Cross plans. In addition, 23 million were served by intermediary contracts with Medicare, Medicaid, and CHAMPUS. (The underwritten federal employees are included in the 74 million.) An additional six million elderly citizens supplement their Medicare coverage with complementary coverage in Blue Cross. Total Blue Cross income in 1970 was $10 billion, one-half of it from private sources, the other half from governmental sources. All Blue Cross plans are involved in the administration of Medicare. Thirty-one plans are also involved in the administration of Medicaid.

As a steadily evolving process, controls on costs are attempted through the following devices:

1. Prospective reimbursement of hospitals for services to Blue Cross subscribers. This method puts the hospitals at risk, in that they will absorb any losses from costs in excess of negotiated rates and sharing any savings with the plans. Only a few plans have made serious efforts to introduce prospective reimbursement.
2. Another cost control device is claims and utilization review. Sixty-eight plans have the utilization review plans of individual hospitals on file and make some attempt to see that these mechanisms are used to control utilization.
3. Thirty plans require recertification of the need for hospitalization following specified numbers of days for various diagnoses.
4. Forty-eight plans contribute directly to support areawide planning of hospital facilities.

---

[18]Another step to increase public accountability was taken by Blue Cross plans in October 1973 when they approved a change in Plan Approval Standards under which, as of January 1, 1975, plan boards must consist of a public majority unless not possible under state law.

In 1974, public representation on plan boards averaged 58 percent (68 percent, if one includes citizens who also serve on hospital boards but are not health professionals).

In addition, Blue Cross plans are broadening out-of-hospital benefits such as outpatient services, drugs, dental care, and home care. In 1969 Blue Cross plans paid out more for out-of-hospital services than for inpatient services. The Blue Cross system is also officially supporting the creation of group practice prepayment medical plans, or health maintenance organizations.

Given all these activities of Blue Cross plans aimed at instituting controls and thus strengthening the honest adversary relationship of plans and hospitals, it is apparent that termination of the interlocking directorate of the Blue Cross Association and the American Hospital Association was appropriate and inevitable. The separation took place early in 1972, with apparent smoothness. The Blue Cross Association took over the approval program of the member plans from the American Hospital Association. The split was symbolized visually by the removal of the seal of the AHA from the Blue Cross insignia. The AHA seal was replaced by the silhouette of a stylized human figure in a circle, symbolizing humanity. The Blue Cross system was now more clearly than ever intent on transcending the particular interests of both subscribers and hospitals. It intended to become a voluntary agency for the general public, pushing on all fronts as a countervailing force to the rigidities inherent in government intervention and in provider institutions protected by licensure and professional tradition. Obviously, the Blue Cross system cannot play this role without hospital rapport; its primary commodity is still hospital service. Thus the relationship is a constantly evolving one. McNerney is well aware of this. In his report to the annual meeting of member plans when the Blue Cross Association and the American Hospital Association separated, he said:

> The realignment of relationships with A.H.A. has left some uncertainty as to what the new relationship should be between member plans and their participating hospitals. The advent of audit review, utilization systems and other control or incentive ventures has caused some hospitals and their associations to view Blue Cross as just another adversary, or as an intermediary with government leanings; but ... keep in mind that hospitals and Blue Cross are the prime community agencies involved in the voluntary sector. Effective communications must continue among them.
>
> There are many forces in operation now that add little to choice and much to non-productive fragmentation—such as certain types of [medical] foundations, PSRO networks [to monitor physician decisions] and free standing institutions. The health field will continue to need a core with a community-oriented conscience. And the fact remains that the hospital is the most promising center for community health.[19]

[19] President's Report, Part I, Annual Meeting of Member Plans, Chicago, Illinois, April 12, 1972.

At the same meeting, recognizing that rapid growth in enrollment was not a realistic expectation, McNerney admonished: "It is not a time for rapid growth in number, but rather a time for identity." The identity is still in formation, and its probable nature will become clearer in a few years.

Further evidence of an emerging new national-local structure for Blue Cross is seen in the report of the annual meeting of the member plans a year later, in May 1973. A great deal of McNerney's report was based on the possibility of some kind of national health insurance program being enacted in the near future. He suggested that the basic character of a national health insurance program would stem from economic considerations, i.e., cost of services, cost controls, competition, and options in delivery systems, rather than from orthodoxies of either the extreme right or left. Those extremes will cancel each other out, he predicted: "The country will buy neither egalitarianism nor elitism. Inequality will be accepted as long as minimum standards are being met and lead to a greater whole." The report continued: "The relative simplicities of the 1960s are over, when Blue Cross could get along by setting competitive rates, paying bills promptly, and having a reasonable benefit package, while stressing good service and fighting to maintain a community orientation as we understand it." The current situation, as described in the report, dictates that Blue Cross must understand in great depth "the political process; the whole strategy of incentives and controls; economic theory and public utility concepts; more complex technology, e.g., data processing and management of larger, more professional, increasingly younger, better educated staffs. And we must act and speak out across a broader spectrum of fronts. Many of us have. Several [plan] presidents, for example, have been explicit about overbuilding of beds or misguided state actions."

As a finishing flourish to inspire the presidents of member plans, McNerney said: ". . . we have a superb format: non-profit, community orientation, ability to move locally or nationally, reflecting the needs of communities, states, or the nation; we are decentralized enough to be managerially sound, yet able to avoid inventing the wheel over and over again through coordination of effort, ability to straddle geographical areas and regions and put together new forms, e.g., HMOs, utilization review, etc., and to weld disparate forces together for better continuity of care; a diverse repository of technical and managerial skills; and excellent communicators with key elements (public and private) in the health system."

This "superb format" was quantified by the following data on Blue Cross system personnel in 1973:

Officers	1,020
Managers	6,480

Professionals	6,540
Technicians	8,700
Sales representatives	3,600
Clerical/service	33,660
Total work force	60,000

Further there are almost 2,000 members of boards of directors of member Blue Cross plans. If unpaid hospital trustees are regarded as public representatives, Blue Cross argues that 68 percent of the members of the boards of directors are public representatives. Seven states—Colorado, Massachusetts, New Jersey, New York, Ohio, Rhode Island, and Virginia—require that a majority of the boards of directors be public. The trend is clearly toward more public representation. The issue then is the legitimacy of this type of representation as really representing the general public. In any case, the Blue Cross system is obviously attempting to strengthen its stance as a community agency. As an effective community agency Blue Cross plans need leverage not only by community composition of its board of directors and contractual relationships with hospitals, but also through the income hospitals receive from Blue Cross in relation to other sources—private insurance and government. Areas vary considerably in the proportions of income hospitals receive from Blue Cross plans, from 15 percent in southern California to 80 percent in Rhode Island. Blue Cross strength lies in New England, the East, and Middle West. These are strong regions economically and politically. A stronger Blue Cross base on the West Coast would be a great help. Still, a Blue Cross plan does not need a majority of the enrollment in an area to be a community force.

The contractual relationship with hospitals strengthens Blue Cross plans considerably and also gives the hospitals some negotiating leverage. This relationship was strengthened further by a court decision late in 1973, after several years of litigation. Private insurance companies for years have resented the position that the hospitals have taken toward Blue Cross plans as a result of contract negotiations. Charges to plans are somewhat lower than charges to subscribers who receive indemnities, because of many factors such as savings on indigent care and bad debts, costs of resident training programs, cash flow, depreciation, and capital requirements. Private insurance companies have felt the contract between hospitals and Blue Cross plans is a form of discriminatory pricing and therefore constitutes unfair competition and restraint of trade.

Travelers Insurance Company brought suit against Blue Cross of Western Pennsylvania (Pittsburgh). This suit went all the way to the Supreme Court, and the decisions were favorable to the Blue Cross plan at all levels. The lower court ruled that the plan's conduct did not violate the antitrust laws; the state regulates the arrangements, the court pointed out, and the economic inducements which made the Blue Cross contract acceptable to hospitals did not amount to coercion, because the hospitals negotiated jointly and the resulting contract was approved by the State Insurance Department.[20]

The Blue Cross system is increasingly and visibly active in supporting what are regarded as progressive actions now taking place in the health services economy in order to control costs and increase accountability. The Blue Cross system supports the concept of utilization review of hospital admissions required by the Medicare Act and is helpful in data processing. Blue Cross is implementing the concept of Professional Standards Review Organizations (PSRO) designed to assure quality and control utilization on an areawide basis. PSROs may well move into home and office visits, as well as hospital service. It is thus apparent that Blue Cross is trying to influence the health services delivery system. Blue Cross also favors certificate-of-need regulations to control the number of hospital beds; 20-odd states have now enacted this type of regulation. Blue Cross is trying to act as a spearhead for the development of various types of comprehensive medical prepayment plans which set up mechanisms for surveillance of physicians' practices to control overprescribing and other improper practices. The popular designation for this type of medical prepayment plan is Health Maintenance Organization (HMO). The Blue Cross–Blue Shield designation for it is "alternative delivery systems."

Since 1970, there has been an impressive increase in alternative delivery systems in which Blue Cross–Blue Shield plans are active. As of November 1973, 34 alternative delivery systems were in operation in 17 cities from California to New York. Three more systems were in the stage of implementation, 13 were being developed, 15 were in the planning stage, and 14 were in the stage of serious investigation. To relate these activities to the Blue Cross plans, 56 plans are involved in the various stages of activity, and 21 plans are involved in prepaid group practice plans in operation. In summary, Blue Cross plans are associated with one-half the prepaid group practice plans in operation.[21]

The Blue Cross system adopted in May 1974 what it called a strategy for cost containment. This statement is in essence a codification and synthesis of evolving cost containment mechanisms, from types of benefit packages to prospective reimbursement with an underpinning of community planning for adequate hospital beds, control of capital budgets, and careful utilization review

[20]Travelers Insurance Company v. Blue Cross of Western Pennsylvania (U.S.Court of Appeals, 3rd Cir., No. 72–1209, July 10, 1973), and Blue Cross Association, *Legal Affairs*, Special Bulletin, Issue no. 189, July 16, 1973.
[21]Blue Cross Association, Health Care Services, Blue Cross and Blue Shield Activity in Alternative Delivery Systems, November 1, 1973.

of admissions and length of stay. The statement was prepared by staff persons who understood the systems nature of the health services delivery mechanism—insofar as it is understood at all. Interesting distinctions are made, for example, between "pressurizing tools" and "venting tools" for cost control. An example of a "pressurizing tool" is claims screening for medical necessity; and an example of a "venting tool" is expansion of out-of-hospital services.

The prevailing opinion currently, as revealed in legislative proposals, is that all these activities are in the public interest in order to control costs, increase delivery system options, and de-emphasize any presumed casual use of the hospital. The Blue Cross system is trying to be a catalyst for the entire health services system.

Thus the Blue Cross system would seem to be poised for developments in the decade ahead. It has the corporate structure, a national organization, experience, and member plans in all states. It has the national communications apparatus to facilitate daily the millions of communications necessary for national and local accounts, a communications system predating Medicare. Important as the structural and organizational aspects of Blue Cross are, the crucial element will continue to be leadership willing to push on the delivery system so that it is open and responsive. From all evidence, this leadership is active in health-related community affairs as well as other community activities.[22] If it is true that hospitals and Blue Cross are the prime community agencies involved in the voluntary sector, the leadership must continue to be both a participant in the mainstream of American health services development and partly detached from it.

[22]Survey of community activities of plan directors, 1974, carried out by Singsen at the suggestion of the writer.

Chapter Eleven

Blue Cross and the Outlook
for National Health Insurance

In 1974, the burning question for Blue Cross has been: What will be our role in the national health insurance program that seems certain to be enacted within the next year or two? As the Congress, through the Ways and Means Committee of the House of Representatives and the Finance Committee of the Senate, considered the dozen or so proposals ranging all the way from a comprehensive government plan supported by tax funds and administered by the Social Security Administration to mandated, privately underwritten catastrophic or major medical insurance at one end of the economic spectrum and subsidies to insure the poor at the other end, there was mounting pressure on the Blue Cross Association to take a position for or against the various bills.

The association felt there was nothing to be gained, however, by supporting or opposing any specific legislative proposal whose provisions, obviously, would undergo substantial changes in the processes of congressional study and consideration. Instead, Blue Cross should emphasize legislation, and the experience and capability Blue Cross would bring to any system.

The concept is to build on what is strong in today's system and evolve the new program in manageable steps. Health should be a concern of all three sectors of our society—government, nonprofit institutions, and proprietary institutions. In joining them together the country can capitalize on the considerable worth of each in order to weld public accountability and institutional independence.

Although any mention of specific legislation is avoided, McNerney does not hesitate to take a position on the goals: "We support the continuation of Medicare as a federally administered program," he declared.[1]

[1] Statement before the House Ways and Means Committee, Washington, D.C., May 3, 1974.

We see the need for a federalized program to serve low income groups. Goals and standards should be clearly enunciated by the federal government. States should be involved only under clearly formulated and approved state plans. Contracts with carriers should benefit from the recommendations of the National Academy of Public Administration [see pp. 2]. The concept of government assistance to individuals or families related to income is sound for both community and individual reasons. We feel that all other persons, most of whom are self-supporting, can be included in national health insurance by capitalizing on the best of private financing mechanisms, including their reimbursement, incentive and control programs, rather than through creating new government agencies. We do not feel that the structure of a trust fund into which many billions of dollars would be channeled is practicable or desirable. . . . Experience teaches us that complex social services are best implemented by focusing on goals while retaining flexibility of means. The myriad technical and professional details involved in health services could evoke an administrative mechanism of endless dimensions if form rather than substance or output became dominant. The public is wary of both big government and big business and not ready to choose up sides.[2]

While McNerney was declaring principles and describing goals and structures for consideration by legislators, he at the same time was adjuring Blue Cross plan executives to shape up for the trial that was obviously going to come. Compared to the Blue Cross state of preparedness at the onset of Medicare in 1966, the plans were told, "The Blue Cross system today is far stronger and in a much better position to handle whatever market or national health insurance requirements are placed upon us."[3] Among the strengths of the system enumerated were the plans' significantly larger and more sophisticated staffs, improved management, programs for monitoring and increasing productivity and efficiency, sophisticated data processing systems, a telecommunications network that had reduced unit cost 25 percent in three years in the face of rising inflation, and broadly expanded Blue Cross subscriber benefits, notably including coverage of ambulatory services.

Touching on a topic that has remained tender throughout Blue Cross history, as this account has indicated, McNerney reminded the plans that in the eyes of subscribers and the public Blue Cross and Blue Shield are perceived as a single entity:

[2]Ibid.
[3]President's Report, Annual Meeting of Blue Cross Plans, San Francisco, California, May 21, 1974.

Nowhere is this perception stronger than it is in the expectations and demands on our systems as they are being expressed today by legislators, public program officials, union and consumer representatives and others whose impact on public policy decisions can bear importantly on our future roles. As the new alternative delivery systems emerge and demonstrate how institutional and professional services can be combined under one point of control, pressures will tend to accentuate for a program relationship among all health care providers. In our marketing, delivery and service programs, a single point of accountability will increasingly be demanded for all health service benefits. For all these reasons, the Blue Cross and Blue Shield systems must be understood on both sides to be interdependent. The problems of one directly reflect and impact upon the other. Relationship and performance problems must be clearly identified and corrected. Public accountability demands it.[4]

Because national health insurance is certain to bring additional pressures to hold down health care costs, and especially hospital costs, the plans need to step up their cost containment efforts as described.

The cost containment strategy of the Blue Cross system is based on moves to (1) shift the demand for the most expensive methods of delivering health care—acute hospital care services—to more economical ways of providing comparable health services while (2) increasing the supply of these more cost-efficient services and (3) increasing the efficiency of all forms of service.

Tools being used by Blue Cross plans to implement this strategy— and contain costs—include utilization review, reimbursement techniques, area-wide planning, public accountability, hospital management programs, benefit expansion, and alternate delivery systems.

To assure that the length of hospital stays and the provision of all health services to patients are medically necessary and appropriate for the diagnosis, utilization review committees are increasingly becoming a Blue Cross plan requirement for facilities providing health care to its subscribers.

Twenty-four plans now have such a requirement and are assisting the committees by furnishing them with useful data on admissions, lengths of stay, and services in comparable hospitals.

The Blue Cross system also has developed a potential cost savings program called Plan Utilization Review (PUR) to encourage and assist plans and their participating institutions to create new, or to improve existing, utilization

[4]Ibid.

review procedures through a sophisticated, computerized screening procedure that checks all claims.

PUR is operating in nine plans and by the end of 1974 was expected to be in operation in at least 17 plans. Forty other plans were doing exploratory work aimed at developing similar programs.

In their work to improve hospitals' internal utilization review programs, Blue Cross plans are sharing their health care data with hospitals. The data are also being shared with Professional Standard Review Organizations (PSROs) for use in medical audits and utilization review.

In a further effort to guard against long hospitalizations, several plans have recertification programs requiring attending physicians to recertify the need for continued hospitalization after a specific time period such as 14 or 21 days (this depending on the nature of treatment provided the patient). Within the next five years it was expected that all Blue Cross plans would have such programs.

Blue Cross plans, over the years, have experimented with new methods of paying hospitals. The method of payment is determined locally through negotiations between a plan and its member hospitals. Guidelines approved by the Blue Cross Association board of governors provide valuable reference points for these negotiations. Traditionally, most hospitals have been paid on the basis of either their costs or negotiated charges. Furthermore, plans conduct or arrange for audits of providers to (1) verify that the costs were incurred and (2) confirm the methods of cost allocations.

In recent years, however, there has been a significant shift to the prospective payment method of reimbursement. Under this method, amounts to be paid to a hospital for various services are determined in advance through negotiations between the hospital and the Blue Cross plan. Financial incentives and possible penalties are included to encourage management and other hospital efficiency.

In 1974, 15 plans representing more than 30 percent of the system's subscribers had some kind of prospective payment method, eight plans were experimenting with it on a limited basis, and another five plans had the method in various stages of program development.

To help assure that needed services are available, the Blue Cross system, nationally and locally, has been one of the earliest supporters of areawide planning. The strength of the system's commitment to areawide planning is seen in the fact that 33 Blue Cross plans have planning-conformance clauses in their hospital contracts, tying reimbursement to areawide planning decisions.

Thirty-one plans are based in the 23 states with certificate of need laws, which are supported by the Blue Cross system and require hospitals to secure permission of an approved state agency to build additional facilities.

More than 80 percent of all Blue Cross subscribers are served by plans which either have planning-conformance clauses in their contracts or are located in certificate of need states. Also, Blue Cross plans contribute to areawide planning agencies as well as providing manpower and data to assist the agencies in their work.

Since public disclosure is at the heart of public accountability—and its impact on greater efficiency and cost savings—the Blue Cross system believes that all aspects of a hospital's performance should be evaluated periodically in the public arena. Accordingly, in November 1973 the Blue Cross Association board issued, as a guideline to the plans, a policy statement to the effect that "health care institutions shall fully disclose the results of their operations to the public and shall undergo independent financial audits which shall also be fully disclosed to the public." In the following year, 29 plans had adopted the provision of the statement requiring independent financial audit and five plans had adopted the statement in full.

Also in November 1973 the BCA board had approved a statement to the effect that "health care institutions should be governed by a board of trustees that is both responsive to, and reasonably representative of, the community that it serves." In 1974 this guideline had been adopted by 14 plans.

Another step to increase public accountability was taken by Blue Cross plans in October 1973 when they approved a change in Plan Approval Standards under which, as of January 1, 1975, plan boards must consist of a public majority unless not possible under state law.

Through cooperative ventures with the hospitals they serve, Blue Cross plans have been in the forefront of many efforts to help control costs by providing hospitals with the tools and techniques to improve management efficiency and productivity.

Examples of these programs include CASH (Commission for Administrative Services in Hospitals), established in 1963 by the Los Angeles plan and a group of southern California hospitals to improve productivity of personnel and the quality of patient care; TEMP (Tennessee Effective Management Program), co-sponsored by the Chattanooga plan and the state hospital association for 23 participating hospitals; PAR (Performance Analysis and Review) which the Pittsburgh plan began in 1969 to utilize management engineering techniques in evaluating productivity in the various hospital departments; and a Maryland plan program of cost verification studies in 45 hospitals.

Also, in Oregon, Washington, and Idaho, the three state Blue Cross plans worked together to finance a program called Systems Program for Hospitals in cooperation with the W. K. Kellogg Foundation and 40 participating hospitals.

Through labor reduction programs, departmental staffing programs, redesign and rescheduling of medical-surgical units, improved methods programs, and other work to improve hospital effectiveness and efficiency, cost savings have been realized through programs such as those cited.

In addition, plans play a significant and growing role as a major supplier of computer services in the health field. The primary concern of plans in providing these services has been to reduce the costs of hospital data processing through the use of shared systems. In 1974 more than 20 plans were engaged in such activities and the Blue Cross Association was giving increasing support to these efforts.

Blue Cross plans have been taking steps in recent years to expand the benefits they offer subscribers, providing coverage of appropriate, lower cost health care services. Expansion has occurred in areas such as out-of-hospital prescription drugs, dental care, treatment of nervous and mental disorders, home care, services in nursing homes and other extended care facilities, and outpatient and preadmission diagnostic services.

As a result, Blue Cross plans now pay more ambulatory claims than impatient claims. During 1973, ambulatory claims paid totalled 13.9 million as compared to 8.6 million claims for hospital admissions.

A few highlights of the benefit expansion program have been:

1. More than two-thirds of all plans had coverage for outpatient X-rays and lab tests;
2. Preadmission testing (PAT) programs were provided as a benefit by 57 plans to 47.7 million persons, making it possible for a patient to get X-ray lab tests in the outpatient department several days before he is actually admitted for surgery or treatment;
3. To further free hospital beds, at least 45 plans had coverage for same-day surgery;
4. Fifty-four plans had 35.7 million persons covered for home care, so a convalescing patient receives in his home a wide range of hospital services and supplies at the fraction of the cost of a hospital day;
5. Sixty-seven plans offer coverage of out-of-hospital drugs;
6. Twenty-nine plans provided dental care coverage.

Commenting on these current efforts, McNerney said, "Blue Cross has come a long way from recertification, audit of costs, negotiated payment formulas and other early control programs. Most plans have made an even-handed attempt to balance subscriber and provider problems in the interest of the community. Now, however, the tempo must be increased. National health insurance, inevitably, will impose some requirements we are not ready to meet in all plans."

While McNerney had discussed Blue Cross performance and readiness chiefly as they related to existing government programs like Medicare and federal employees benefits and, especially, the expected onset of national health insurance, he considered that precisely the same elements could appropriately have been listed even if national health insurance was not in sight. The complexities obviously multiply with the growing fraction of services that are paid for by government and thus necessarily measured and monitored by law and regulatory authority, but the basic tasks of serving subscribers, dealing fairly with providers and sources of funding, and maintaining the required equilibrium of these often divergent interests and forces are the same, whatever the populations and programs.

Thus Blue Cross in 1974 was expanding on the same principles and goals that had been articulated by Rorem 40 years earlier, a unique performance for social institutions in our time. Clearly, this country contains the elements of a viable pluralistic system for health services—if there is enough political sophistication to structure the relationships.

Appendix A

LIST OF INTERVIEWS BY THE WRITER

Abbot, Charles—Los Angeles, California, April 25, 1973
Ball, Robert—Washington, D.C., November 14, 1973
Barham, Sam—Topeka, Kansas, April 22, 1973
Beauchamp, Tom L.—Dallas, Texas, May 3, 1972
Bennett, T. B.—Baton Rouge, Louisiana, August 29, 1972
Bethel, Ralph—Tulsa, Oklahoma, April 24, 1973
Blair, A.G.—Edmonton, Alberta, Canada, March 19, 1972
Brockway, Richard—New York, New York, August 28, 1973
Brown, Harold—Montreal, Quebec, Canada, June 19, 1973
Buerki, Robin, M.D.—Chicago, Illinois, April 17, 1972
Bugbee, George—Genesee Depot, Wisconsin, March 17, 1971
Cahalane, Reginald—Walpole, New Hampshire, August 5, 1971
Cannon, Walter E.—Chicago, Illinois, August 22, 1973
Castellucci, John—Ft. Lauderdale, Florida, March 23, 1973
Clark, Kenneth—Rockford, Illinois, December 19, 1972
Colman, J. Douglas—New York, New York, January 9, 1971
Crawford, E.B.—Chapel Hill, North Carolina, May 21, 1971
Crownhart, Charles H.—Madison, Wisconsin, August 10, 1972
Davis, Michael M.—Chevy Chase, Maryland, February 7, 1971
Dickson, Frank—Portland, Oregon, April 30, 1972
Doyle, T. Ledwell—Montreal, Quebec, Canada, June 19, 1973
Durgom, J. Albert—Chicago, Illinois, January 3, 1973
Falk, I. S.—New Haven, Connecticut, April 2, 1971
Feierabend, F. L., M.D.—Kansas City, Missouri, August 31, 1971
Fletcher, Abbot—Minneapolis, Minnesota, August 12, 1972
Ford, William H.—O'Hare Airport, Chicago, Illinois, March 28, 1973
Green, Gerry M.—Chicago, Illinois, June 5, 1973
Guy, William—Los Angeles, California, April 25, 1973

Heitler, George—Chicago, Illinois, June 12, 1973
Jones, Richard M.—Portland, Oregon, April 30, 1972
Kammer, Earl E.—Cincinnati, Ohio, November 30, 1972
Ketchum, Jay—Ft. Lauderdale, Florida, March 23, 1973
Kretchmer, C. J.—Seattle, Washington, May 1, 1971
Lattner, Fritz—Des Moines, Iowa, December 6, 1972
McCue, W. A.—Bluefield, West Virginia, November 3, 1971
McMahon, John Alexander—Chicago, Illinois, August 2, 1973
McNary, William S.—Detroit, Michigan, July 30, 1971
McNerney, Walter J.—Chicago, Illinois, June 13, 1973
Mannix, John—Cleveland, Ohio, February 24, 1971
Maybee, Harold—Wilmington, Delaware, November 14, 1973.
Millican, Duncan—Montreal, Quebec, Canada, June 19, 1973
Nelson, J. Philo—San Francisco, California, April 7, 1971
Norby, Maurice J.—Deerfield, Illinois, September 14, 1971
Offerman, Arthur J., M.D.—Omaha, Nebraska, March 26, 1971
O'Leary, Albert—St. Paul Minnesota, August 12, 1972
Pearce, Harold—Chicago, Illinois, June 11, 1973
Reed, Louis S.—McLean, Virginia, February 7, 1971
Rorem, C. Rufus—New York, New York, December 17, 1970
Schroder, H.A.—Jacksonville, Florida, March 22, 1973
Sibery, D. Eugene—Chicago, Illinois, June 12, 1973
Singleton, H. F.—Birmingham, Alabama, June 1, 1972
Singsen, Antone G.—Chicago, Illinois, June 28, 1973
Suycott, Leo E.—Milwaukee, Wisconsin, August 9, 1972
Taylor, Bruce—Philadelphia, Pennsylvania, June 11, 1973
Tresnowski, Bernard—Chicago, Illinois, September 7, 1973
Vallon, E. J.—New Orleans, Louisiana, November 8, 1972
Van Dyk, Frank—New York, New York, May 11, 1971
van Steenwyk, John—Chicago, Illinois, August 21, 1973
Walker, Marvin—Cincinnati, Ohio, November 30, 1972
Webb, Paul—Falmouth, Maine, August 7, 1971
Werner, Edwin R.—New York, New York, February 27, 1974

Appendix B

**INTERVIEWS CONDUCTED BY THE BLUE CROSS
COMMISSION IN CONNECTION WITH THE
25TH ANNIVERSARY OF BLUE CROSS, 1954**

Groner, Edward—New Orleans, Louisiana, December 27
Helland, N.D.—Tulsa, Oklahoma, August 12
Kimball, Justin F.—Dallas, Texas, August 6
Payne, Lawrence—Tyler, Texas, August 19
Twitty, Bryce—Tulsa, Oklahoma, August 12
Van Dyk, Frank—Chicago, Illinois, July 23
van Steenwyk, E. A.—Philadelphia, Pennsylvania, July 28

Appendix C

LOCAL BLUE CROSS HISTORIES

Breed, William C. *History of Associated Hospital Service of New York*. New York: The Associated Hospital Service, 1959.

Clark, Kenneth. *The History of Rockford Blue Cross*. Unpublished, no date.

Fletcher, Abbot Lee *History of Minnesota Blue Cross*. No publisher, no date.

Gibson, Ernest R. *A Quarter Century of Progress; A History of Blue Cross in Florida, 1944–1969*. Jacksonville, Florida: Blue Cross of Florida, 1969.

Henryson, E. J. *My Story of Group Hospitalization, Inc*. Washington, D.C.: Kaufman/Graphiss, 1971?

Nelson, R.W. *Origin and Development of the Blue Cross Plan in Oregon and the Pacific Northwest*. Unpublished, no date. (latter 1960s?)

Pennsylvania Economy League, Inc. *The Middle Road; An Evaluation of Blue Cross Service; A Report Based on a Study of the Hospital Service Association of Western Pennsylvania*. Pittsburgh: The Association, 1959?

Sinclair, Frank. *Blue Cross in Wisconsin*. Milwaukee: Blue Cross 1965.

Taylor, Robert D. *Plan History* (Western Pennsylvania) 1968. Typewritten manuscript.

Bibliography

American Hospital Association. *Transactions of the 33rd Annual Convention*. Toronto, Ontario, Canada, September 28–October 2, 1931.

Andersen, Ronald and Anderson, Odin W. *A Decade of Health Services; Social Survey Trends in Use and Expenditures*. Chicago: University of Chicago Press, 1967.

Anderson, Odin W. *Health Care: Can There Be Equity? The United States, Sweden, and England*. New York: John Wiley & Sons, Inc., 1972

——.*State Enabling Legislation for Non-Profit Hospital and Medical Plans, 1944*. School of Public Health, Public Health Economics, Research Series No. 1. Ann Arbor: University of Michigan, 1944.

——. *The Uneasy Equilibrium; Private and Public Financing of Health Services in the United States, 1875–1965*. New Haven, Connecticut: College and University Press, 1968.

Anderson, Odin W. and May, J. Joel. *The Federal Employees Health Benefits Program: 1961–1968; A Model for National Health Insurance?* Perspectives A9. Chicago: Center for Health Administration Studies, University of Chicago, 1971.

Ball, Robert M. "That Illusive Partnership." Speech delivered before the Colorado Hospital Association, Aspen, Colorado, September 13, 1973.

Blue Cross Association. Minutes of annual meetings from its inception to date.

——. *The Blue Cross Story*. Chicago: 1972.

——. *Legal Affairs*. Special Bulletin, Issue no. 189. Chicago, July 16, 1973.

Blue Cross Association and American Hospital Association, Joint Committee. *Financing Health Care of the Aged*. Pts. I and II. Chicago: 1962.

Blue Cross Commission. Minutes of annual meetings from 1936 (including the Commission predecessors).

Blumberg, Phillip I. "The Politicization of the Corporation." *The Business Lawyer*, July 1971, pp. 1551–87.

Boorstin, Daniel J. *The Genius of American Politics*. Chicago: University of Chicago Press, 1953.

Brush, Frederick, M.D. Transactions of the American Hospital Association, 11th Annual Conference XI, 1909.

Committee for Economic Development. Research and Policy Committee. *Social Responsibilities of Business Corporations; A Statement on National Policy*. New York: 1971.

Cunningham, Robert M. *The Blue Cross Story*. 2nd ed. New York: Public Affairs Committee, 1963. (1st ed., 1958)

Dahl, Robert A. *Pluralistic Democracy in the United States—Conflict and Consent*. Chicago: Rand McNally, 1967.

Dahl, Robert A. and Lindblom, Charles E. *Politics, Economics and Welfare*. New York: Harper, 1953.

DeGré, Girard. "Freedom and Social Structure." *American Sociological Review*, 11 (October 1946): 529–36.

DeWitt, Benjamin Parke. *The Progressive Movement; A Non-Partisan, Comprehensive Discussion of Current Tendencies in American Politics*. Seattle: University of Washington Press, 1968.

Friedman, Milton. *Capitalism and Freedom*. Chicago: University of Chicago Press, 1963.

Harris, Louis. *The Anguish of Change*. New York: Norton, 1973.

Heyne, Paul T. *Private Keepers of the Public Interest*. New York: McGraw-Hill, 1968.

Hofstadter, Richard. *The Age of Reform from Bryan to FDR*. New York: Knopf, 1955.

Jacoby, Neil H. *Corporate Power and Social Responsibility; A Blueprint for the Future*. New York: MacMillan, 1973.

Lerner, Monroe and Anderson, Odin W. *Health Progress in the United States: 1900–1960*. Chicago: University of Chicago Press, 1963.

Levin, Sol; Anderson, Odin W.; and Gordon, Gerald. *Non-Group Enrollment for Health Insurance; A Study of Administrative Approaches of Blue Cross Plans*. Cambridge, Massachusetts: Harvard University Press, 1957.

Lindblom, Charles E. *The Intelligence of Democracy: Decision-Making Through Mutual Adjustment*. New York: Free Press, 1965.

Lippmann, Walter. *The Good Society: An Inquiry into the Principles of a Good Society*. New York: Little, Brown and Co., 1937.

Lowi, Theodore. *The End of Liberalism: Ideology, Policy, and the Crisis of Public Authority*. New York: Norton, 1969.

MacIntyre, Duncan M. *Voluntary Health Insurance and Rate Making*. Ithaca, New York: Cornell University Press, 1962.

McNerney, Walter J. Statement before Subcommittee on Anti-Trust and Monopoly, U.S. Senate. Washington, D.C. January 28, 1971.

McNerney, Walter J. and Study Staff. *Hospital and Medical Economics: A Study of Population, Services, Costs, Methods of Payment, and Controls*. 2 vols. Chicago: Hospital Research and Educational Trust, 1962.

Mannix, John R. "Prepayment, Hospitals and the Future; Needed: Strong Leadership and a Unified Blue Cross." *Hospitals*, November 1, 1959. (Reprint.)

———. "Why Not an American Blue Cross?" *Hospitals*, April, 1944. (Reprint.)

Marmor, Theodore R. with Marmor, Jan S. *The Politics of Medicare*. London, England: Routledge and Kegan Paul, 1970.

Mowry, George E. *The California Progressives*. Berkeley: University of California Press, 1951.

National Academy of Public Administration. *Final Report of the Medicare Project Panel*. Washington, D.C.: June 30, 1973.

National Health Council. *The Changing Role of the Public and Private Sectors in Health Care*. Report of the 1973 National Health Forum. New York: 1973.

Pink, Louis H. *The Story of Blue Cross; On the Road to Better Health*. New York: Public Affairs Committee, 1945.

The President's Commission on the Health Needs of the Nation. *Building America's Health: Findings and Recommendations*. 5 vols. 1952.

Reed, Louis S. *Blue Cross and Medical Services Plans*. Washington, D.C.: Federal Security Agency, Public Health Service, 1947.

— —. *Health Insurance: The Next Step in Social Security*. New York: Harper, 1937.

Rittel, Horst W. J. and Webber, Melvin M. "Dilemmas in a General Theory of Planning." *Policy Sciences* 4, (1973): 155–69.

Robinson, David Z. "Government Contracting for Academic Research: Accountability in the American Experience," *In The Dilemma of Public Accountability in Modern Government*. Bruce L. R. Smith and D. C. Hague, eds. New York: St. Martin's Press, 1971.

Rorem, C. Rufus. "Hospital Care a Community Affair: The Justin Ford Kimball Award Address." Blue Cross Program Session, April 13, 1959.

———. "The New Philadelphia Blue Cross Hospital Agreement; Milestone or Millstone?" Unpublished, 1973.

———. *The Public's Investment in Hospitals*. Chicago: University of Chicago Press, 1930.

Rose, Arnold. *The Power Structure: Political Process in American Society*. New York: Oxford, 1967.

Skidmore, Max J. *Medicare and the American Rhetoric of Reconciliation*. University, Alabama: University of Alabama Press, 1970.

Smith, Bruce L. R. "Accountability and Independence in the Contract State," *In The Dilemma of Accountability in Modern Government; Independence Versus Contract*. Bruce L. R. Smith and D. C. Hague, eds. New York: St. Martin's Press, 1971.

Smith, Bruce L. R. and Hollander, Neil, eds. *The Administration of Medicare: A Shared Responsibility*. Washington, D.C.: National Academy of Public Administration, 1973.

Somers, Herman M. and Somers, Anne R. *Medicare and the Hospitals; Issues and Prospects*. Washington, D.C.: Brookings Institution, 1967.

Stuart, James E. "Blue Cross Slips Are Showing," *Modern Hospital*, August, 1953, 1–2. (Reprint.)

———. "The Blue Cross History: An Informal Biography of the Voluntary Non-Profit Prepayment Plan for Hospital Care." Unpublished manuscript, 1966.

Sundquist, James L. *Dynamics of the Party System: Alignment and Realignment of Political Parties in the United States*. Washington, D.C.: Brookings Institution, 1973.

———. *Politics and Policy: The Eisenhower, Kennedy and Johnson Years*. Washington, D.C.: Brookings Institution, 1968.

Travelers Insurance Co. v. Blue Cross of Western Pennsylvania. U.S. Court of Appeals, 3rd Cir., No. 72–1209, July 10, 1973.

"The Truman Memories." *Life*, XL, (January 23, 1956): 104.

U.S. Federal Security Agency. *The Nation's Health; A Ten-Year Program: A Report to the President*. Washington, D.C.: 1948.

Van Dyk, Frank. "A Group Hospital Insurance Plan." *Bulletin of the American Hospital Association*, 7 (January 1933): 45–60.

van Steenwyk, John. "Blue Cross—A Nationwide Hospital Service System." MBA thesis in insurance, Graduate Division of the Wharton School, University of Pennsylvania, 1955 (Typewritten).

Wiebe, Robert H. *The Search for Order, 1877–1920*. The Making of America Series. New York: Hill and Wang, 1967.

Wildavsky, Aaron. *The Politics of the Budgetary Process*. Boston: Little, Brown and Co., 1964.

Wilensky, Harold L. and Lebeaux, Charles N. *Industrial Society and Social Welfare*. New York: Russell Sage Foundation, 1958.

Index

About the Author

Odin W. Anderson Ph.D. (Sociology, University of Michigan) is Professor of Sociology in the Graduate School of Business and the Department of Sociology and Director of the Center for Health Administration Studies, University of Chicago. His major interests lie in the organization and financing of health services and he is the author or co-author of numerous books and articles on these topics. He is a Fellow of the American Sociological Association, American Public Health Association, The Institute of Medicine of the National Science Foundation, and an Honorary Fellow of the American College of Hospital Administrators.